Complementary and Alternative Medicine and Multiple Sclerosis

Second Edition

Complementary and Alternative Medicine and Multiple Sclerosis

Second Edition

Allen C. Bowling, M.D., Ph.D.

Medical Director
The Rocky Mountain Multiple Sclerosis Center
Englewood, Colorado

and

Clinical Associate Professor of Neurology
University of Colorado at Denver and Health Sciences Center
Denver, Colorado

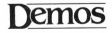

Demos Medical Publishing, LLC, 386 Park Avenue South, New York, New York 10016

Visit our website at www.demosmedpub.com

The first edition of this book was published in 2001 under the title
Alternative Medicine and Multiple Sclerosis.

Library of Congress Cataloging-in-Publication Data

Bowling, Allen C.
    Complementary and alternative medicine and multiple sclerosis
  Allen C. Bowling—2nd ed.
      p. ; cm.
     Rev. ed. of: Alternative medicine and multiple sclerosis. c2001.
    Includes bibliographical references and index.
    ISBN-13: 978-1-932603-54-5 (pbk. : alk. paper)
    ISBN-10: 1-932603-54-9 (pbk. : alk. paper)
    1. Multiple sclerosis—Alternative treatment.   I. Bowling, Allen C.
Alternative medicine and multiple sclerosis. II. Title.
    [DNLM: 1. Multiple Sclerosis—therapy. 2. Complementary
Therapies. WL 360 B787a 2007]
  RC377.B6 2007
  616.8'3406—dc22

                               2006026764

Manufactured in the United States of America
08 09 10 5 4 3 2

To my wife, Diana

Contents

Part 3   *A Five-Step Approach: Integrating Conventional and Unconventional Medicine*

Foreword

$\mathcal{F}$ew areas in medicine raise as much controversy and debate as the use of the wide range of interventions contained under the banner heading of complementary and alternative medicine (CAM). However, it is important from the outset to appreciate that many approaches are grouped under this heading and that they often differ fundamentally from one another. One thing all these approaches do have in common is that they raise great interest and enthusiasm among people with medical conditions, and they are used by many who believe they derive benefit from them.

Taking a more critical view, major differences exist in the quality and quantity of evidence supporting the use of approaches contained within CAM. Furthermore, although such evidence is considered essential by most medical practitioners and those who seek to guide them, it can be less of an issue to those with chronic disabling conditions with no cure and inadequate symptom management. This is precisely the case with multiple sclerosis (MS), a variable condition that may result in progressive disability and cause a plethora of interacting and distressing symptoms. Many of those with MS are prepared to consider any possible remedy, and they certainly want accurate and up-to-date information about all possible therapeutic approaches.

It is, therefore, not surprising that many people with MS have tried at least one (and often many more than one) of the approaches constituting CAM. They require accurate and accessible information, provided in an objective and clear style, to inform and guide their decision to take (or not to take) these treatments. This is precisely what Dr. Allen Bowling has achieved in this comprehensive book on CAM. In his clear and authoritative style, he presents what is currently known on a wide range of potential treatments. He cites evidence where it exists, and discusses treatment options clearly and objectively. His approach is firmly based on his clinical experience and extensive interactions with people with MS. As a result, the book has a clear patient focus. It is an essential resource for people with

MS and for all those who are involved in their care, and it will become an invaluable guide in their joint decision-making.

Alan J. Thompson, MD, FRCP, FRCPI.
Garfield Weston Professor of Clinical Neurology and Rehabilitation
Institute of Neurology
University College London
Clinical Director
National Hospital for Neurology and Neurosurgery
London, United Kingdom

Preface

This book was written to provide accurate and helpful information about complementary and alternative medicine (CAM) to people with multiple sclerosis (MS). The term CAM refers broadly to medical approaches, such as acupuncture or herbal medicine, that are not typical components of conventional medicine. Despite the fact that the majority of people with MS appear to use CAM, it may be difficult to find reliable information about the relevance and usefulness of these therapies in MS. Those who practice a therapy or who are selling products may not understand MS or may exaggerate claims in order to make sales. On the other hand, physicians and other health care professionals often have little or no information or experience in CAM and may not have the resources to provide accurate information to their patients. This book was written to fill the information gap in this area.

The first edition of this book was published in 2001. About four years later, I was told by Dr. Diana Schneider and others at Demos Medical Publishing that a second edition needed to be written and that it was "not a big deal" to write a second edition. After my experiences of the past several months, I would respectfully disagree with this statement. In a way, it is exciting that it was a huge task to write the second edition. This indicates that the area of CAM and MS is dynamic and growing, that new research is underway, and that ongoing interest persists in the subject. Certainly, my own experience indicates that people with MS continue to use and be interested in CAM and that MS health professionals are increasingly interested in and open to discussing the subject.

Providing CAM information has many potential benefits. People with MS may realize that unconventional treatment options may offer relief and hope for situations in which limited conventional medical therapies are available. Providing access to reliable CAM information also should allow people to avoid potentially dangerous interactions between CAM therapies and conventional medicine and to distinguish CAM therapies that are possibly effective, low risk, and inexpensive from those that are ineffective, dangerous, or costly. Finally, it is hoped that the objective information in this book will remove some of the prejudices and misperceptions that are rampant in this area, stimulate serious thought and discussion about CAM and MS, and lead to further study of those therapies that are widely used or appear promising.

This book is divided into three main sections. The first section provides a general introduction to MS and CAM. The second section, which is the main portion of the book, presents detailed information on a large number of CAM modalities. This section is organized alphabetically, which should allow the reader to quickly find information on a particular CAM therapy. The final section includes a chapter that outlines a five-step strategy for integrating conventional and unconventional medicine. At the end of the book, a Glossary of Popular Supplements provides a quick source of MS-relevant information about commonly used supplements.

A large number of references were used to write this book. More than 80 books and more than 2,000 scientific and clinical journal articles were reviewed. The most relevant books and journal articles are listed under an Additional Resources section at the end of the chapters. These resources include technical as well as nontechnical material. In addition, when specific data are mentioned in the text, a numerical reference is given that may be found in a detailed reference section at the end of the book. Most of the books referenced should be available through public libraries, medical libraries, or bookstores. Summaries or abstracts of the journal articles may be found by using Medline searches, available through the website of the National Library of Medicine (www.nlm.nih.gov). The entire articles may be obtained from medical libraries.

Organization of Chapters and Reading Sequence

The second section of this book evaluates many different CAM therapies, which are arranged alphabetically so that they are easy to locate. This arrangement of chapters may be awkward if you intend to read through the entire book. A possibly useful organization and reading sequence is one based on the National Institutes of Health classification for CAM. If this sequence is followed, the structured reading sequence is as follows:

Biologically Based Therapies

Diets—Diets and Fatty Acid Supplements
Herbal Medicine
    Herbs
    Marijuana
    Aromatherapy
Orthomolecular Medicine
    Vitamins, minerals, and other nonherbal supplements
Pharmacologic, Biologic, and Instrumental Interventions
    Allergies
    Aspartame
    Bee venom therapy
    Candida treatment
    Chelation therapy
    Cooling therapy
    Dental amalgam removal
    Enzyme therapy
    Hyperbaric oxygen
    Low-dose naltrexone (LDN)
    Prokarin
    Toxins

Alternative Medical Systems

Acupuncture and Traditional Chinese Medicine
Ayurveda
Homeopathy
T'ai Chi

Lifestyle and Disease Prevention

Exercise

Mind–Body Medicine

Biofeedback
Guided Imagery
Hypnosis
Meditation
Music Therapy
Pets
Prayer and Spirituality
Yoga

Manipulative and Body-Based Systems

Massage and Body Work
    Chiropractic medicine
    Craniosacral therapy
    Feldenkrais
    Massage
    Pilates method
    Reflexology
    Tragerwork
Unconventional Physical Therapies
    Colon therapy
    Hippotherapy and therapeutic horseback riding

Energy Therapies

Magnets and Electromagnetic Therapy
Therapeutic Touch

Acknowledgments

Many individuals and organizations made this book possible. First, I would like to thank my wife, Diana, for her patience and ongoing support. She offered valuable and provocative insight into the subject of CAM. She created time for me to write and provided free psychotherapy during the more challenging times! I thank our two daughters, Elizabeth and Sarah, for tolerating my time away from home, my time working at home, and for teaching me regularly that in daily life, as in medicine, there are many different perspectives on a given situation. I thank all of my family for tolerating late nights, early mornings, laundry baskets piled high with books and files, and counters and tabletops crowded with papers.

This book would not have been possible without the support of the Board of Directors, as well as Karen Wenzel, Executive Director, and other staff at the Rocky Mountain Multiple Sclerosis Center. Dr. Ronald S. Murray encouraged development of this project in the early stages. Thomas Stewart, J.D., PA.-C., M.S., played an important role by devoting time and energy to the research and by providing creative input. Patricia Kennedy, R.N., C.N.P., and Lee Shaughnessy read the initial manuscript carefully and made valuable suggestions. Research assistance was provided by Lee Shaughnessy, Dr. Ragaa Ibrahim, and Julie Lawton for the first edition and by Kathy Haruf for the second edition.

Many of my patients at the MS Center motivated me to write this book. Through my patients, I learned that many were quite devoted to CAM therapies. I realized that I knew little about some of these therapies that obviously were an important component of their health care. I respect my patients for their willingness to openly share their feelings and experiences related to CAM, and I thank them for providing first-hand information that was critical in the development of this book.

I thank the users of www.ms-cam.org, the CAM website of the Rocky Mountain Multiple Sclerosis Center. Users of this website have generously participated in our surveys, which allow us to research the types of CAM that people with MS are using and determine whether these therapies are thought to be helpful or harmful. The results of many of these surveys are included in this book, have been published in lay and professional publications, and have been presented to lay and professional audiences.

A number of organizations and individuals provided valuable advice, information, and financial or moral support: Therese Beaudette, R.D.; my parents, Dr. Franklin Bowling and Ruth Bowling, R.D.; Scott Boynton, DiplAc, B.Ac.; Dr. Jay Schneiders; Joan Wolk and Edith Barry at Demos Medical Publishing; Doris Borchert at the Medical Library at Swedish Medical Center; HealthONE Foundation; Denver Botanic Gardens; Hudson Gardens. Lastly, I thank Dr. Diana M. Schneider at Demos Medical Publishing for her ongoing support, thoughtful input, and willingness to pursue this controversial subject.

Complementary and Alternative Medicine

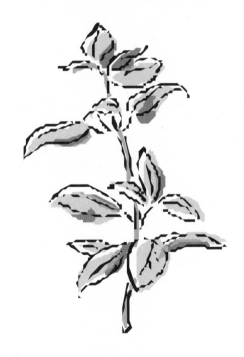

1

Complementary and Alternative Medicine (CAM)

Multiple sclerosis (MS) is a common disease of the nervous system. Most people with MS use some form of conventional medical treatment. In addition, many people with MS also use complementary and alternative medicine (CAM), which refers to unconventional medical practices that are not part of mainstream medicine. Despite the fact that CAM is used frequently and MS is a common neurologic disorder, it may be difficult to obtain accurate and unbiased information specific to the use of CAM for MS.

Before considering the relevance of unconventional medicine to MS, it is important to understand the approach of conventional medicine to this disease. Dramatic advances have occurred recently in the field of MS research. Through scientific studies, we now have an increased understanding of the disease process itself. Also, clinical studies using experimental medications have yielded new therapies that slow the disease process and control MS-related symptoms, such as stiffness or pain.

Who Develops MS?

MS is a common neurologic disease that affects 350,000 to 400,000 people in the United States. Women are diagnosed with the disease about twice as frequently as are men. Although MS may affect people in all age groups, it is typically diagnosed between the ages of 20 and 40 years. A striking relationship exists between the prevalence of MS and the geographic area in which an individual lived during childhood. In general, an individual has a higher risk of developing MS if he or she grew up in an area that is far from the equator and a lower risk if the childhood years were spent near the equator.

3

How Does MS Affect the Nervous System?

In contrast to many diseases that affect a single part of the human body, MS affects two different body systems: the immune system and the nervous system. The immune system is not a distinct organ like the brain or liver. Instead, it is composed of many different types of molecules and cells (known as white blood cells) that travel through the bloodstream. The immune cells use chemical messages to protect the body from attack by bacteria, viruses, and cancers. MS is believed to be an *autoimmune condition* in which the immune system is excessively active and actually attacks the nervous system.

The *central nervous system* (CNS) is the part of the nervous system involved in MS. The CNS includes the brain and spinal cord. The nerves in the CNS communicate with each other through long, wire-like processes that have a central fiber (*axon*) surrounded by an insulating material (*myelin*). In MS, the immune system cells produce inflammation that injures the myelin. In addition, damage occurs to the axon. This damage is known as *degeneration*, which is the process that occurs in aging-related neurologic diseases such as Alzheimer's and Parkinson's disease. The injury to the myelin and axons results in a slowing or blocking of nerve impulses that prevents the affected parts of the nervous system from functioning normally.

The cause of MS is not entirely clear. It is believed that two important factors are involved in developing the disease, one of which is environmental and the other genetic. The characteristic geographic distribution of MS indicates that an environmental factor is present. One hypothesis is that individuals are exposed to a particular virus during childhood. This viral infection may be more common in cooler climates that are more distant from the equator. Another theory relates the geographic distribution to vitamin D, which mildly suppresses the immune system and thus could be protective against MS. Because vitamin D becomes active with sunlight exposure, those who live farther from the equator (with less-direct sunlight exposure) may have lower levels of vitamin D levels and higher risks of developing MS.

The presence of a genetic factor is suggested by family studies that demonstrate a hereditary predisposition to MS. Some genetic diseases are "dominant" and are clearly passed down through generations. MS usually is not passed on in such a well-defined pattern. Rather, there may exist an inherited predisposition to the disease that must be present in addition to an environmental agent to cause disease. Ongoing, intensive research efforts are aimed at identifying specific genes that increase the risk of developing MS or affect the severity of the disease.

What Symptoms Do People with MS Experience?

The symptoms of MS depend on which areas of the brain and spinal cord develop MS *lesions*. For example, if the nerve that is involved in vision (the optic nerve) develops a lesion, blurring of vision occurs. This is referred to as *optic neuritis*. If a lesion develops in the part of the brain that produces movement on the left side of the body, left-sided weakness develops. In addition to visual blurring and weakness, other common MS symptoms include fatigue, depression, urinary difficulties, walking unsteadiness, stiffness in the arms or legs, tingling, and numbness.

The time course over which MS lesions develop and the number and location of lesions is different for each individual. Consequently, the time frame in which symptoms occur and the specific types of symptoms experienced are unique for each person. Also, as a result of the large variability of lesions between individuals, MS varies greatly in severity. Some people may have rare, mild attacks over their lifetime and may not experience any permanent symptoms, whereas others may develop severe, permanent symptoms over a relatively short period.

MS symptoms may occur episodically or may progress continuously. Episodes of symptoms are known as *relapses*, *attacks*, or *exacerbations*. Usually, some improvement in symptoms occurs after an attack. This improvement is referred to as a *remission*. In contrast to these relapsing-remitting symptoms, some people have symptoms that develop slowly and then progressively worsen over time with no clear remissions. These symptoms are referred to as *progressive*.

Specific combinations of relapsing-remitting and progressive symptoms are the basis for classifying MS. People who experience attacks and then improve have *relapsing-remitting MS*. This is the most common type of MS at the time of diagnosis. Some people who initially have relapsing-remitting disease may subsequently develop progressive symptoms. This is known as *secondary-progressive MS*. People who have exclusively progressive symptoms from the onset of the disease, which is relatively rare, have *primary-progressive MS*, whereas those with *progressive-relapsing MS* have progressive symptoms from the onset (as occurs with *primary-progressive MS*), but also experience intermittent relapses.

Conventional Medical Therapy for MS

Dramatic advances have been made recently in the treatment of MS. In the past, no particularly effective therapies were available to change the course of disease.

Since 1993, six medications for MS have been approved by the U.S. Food and Drug Administration (FDA). Four of these are commonly used as initial MS therapies: interferon beta-1b (Betaseron), interferon beta-1a once-weekly (Avonex), interferon beta-1a three-times-weekly (Rebif), and glatiramer acetate (Copaxone). Mitoxantrone (Novantrone) is a chemotherapy medication that is typically used for people who do not respond to the other four medications. Another MS medication known as natalizumab (Tysabri) was approved by the FDA in 2006. These drugs decrease the number and severity of relapses, slow the progression of the disease, and decrease the development of new brain lesions.

Because of the positive effects of the FDA-approved medications, all people with MS should be strongly considered for treatment with one of these drugs. A 1998 statement by the National Multiple Sclerosis Society emphasized the importance of treatment. The statement recommended that treatment with these medications should be started soon after an MS diagnosis is made and should be considered in all people with MS, regardless of age, rate of relapses, and level of disability.

In addition to these medications, several other medications are used to treat MS. Steroids are used for exacerbations. These may be taken orally (prednisone, dexamethasone) or intravenously (methylprednisolone or Solu-Medrol). Some chemotherapy medications other than mitoxantrone, including methotrexate, azathioprine (Imuran), and cyclophosphamide (Cytoxan), occasionally are used in an attempt to slow disease progression.

Given the wide range of symptoms caused by MS, multiple treatment approaches are possible. Therapies for symptoms include medication-based and nonmedication approaches, such as physical therapy, occupational therapy, speech therapy, and psychotherapy. Common MS symptoms that are treated using these therapies include fatigue, depression, weakness, incoordination, walking difficulties, stiffness, bowel and bladder disorders, and sexual difficulties.

(For more information on conventional approaches to MS, see the other, more extensive texts in this area in the "Additional Readings" section at the end of this chapter.)

Complementary and Alternative Medicine

CAM is a controversial area. In fact, even the term and its definition are not entirely agreed on. In addition to complementary and alternative medicine, other frequently used terms are *unconventional medicine and integrative medicine*. The term complementary medicine refers to therapies that are used *in addition* to conventional medicine, while the term alternative medicine is used to describe treatments that are used *instead* of conventional medicine.

CAM has many different definitions. These definitions frequently state what CAM "is not" as opposed to what it "is." For example, in the United States, CAM is sometimes defined as medical therapy that is not widely taught at American medical schools or is not generally available in American hospitals. This definition recently has become less clear because unconventional medicine is now part of the curricula of many medical schools and is available in some medical communities. Also, as clinical trials are done to evaluate the effectiveness of CAM therapies, some forms of CAM may eventually become components of conventional medicine.

CAM includes a vast number of therapies. Multiple schemes have been proposed for categorizing these diverse and often unrelated therapies. A cumbersome yet useful CAM classification scheme has been developed by the National Institutes of Health (NIH). This scheme and some representative examples of therapies are:

- Biologically based therapies—Dietary supplements, diets, bee venom therapy, hyperbaric oxygen
- Mind–body therapies—Guided imagery, hypnosis, meditation
- Alternative medical systems—Traditional Chinese medicine, Ayurveda, homeopathy
- Manipulative and body-based therapies—Chiropractic, reflexology, massage
- Energy therapies—Therapeutic touch, magnets

Several studies have documented that CAM is used frequently in the United States. One well-known large study was conducted in 1997 and was reported in the medical literature in 1998 by Dr. David Eisenberg (1). In this study of more than 2,000 people, approximately 42 percent used some form of CAM. It was estimated that 629 million visits were made to practitioners of alternative medicine; this was greater than the number of visits to all primary care physicians in that year. Nearly 20 percent of people were taking some type of herb or vitamin along with a prescription medication. Most people used CAM without the supervision of a CAM practitioner, and most people did not discuss their use of CAM with their physicians. As a result, nearly half of the people were using CAM without the advice of a physician or a CAM practitioner. This demonstrates the need for increased communication in this area between patients and health care providers.

This 1997 study was a follow-up to a previous study conducted in 1990 (2). From 1990 to 1997, CAM use increased by 25 percent, and the yearly visits to CAM practitioners increased by 47 percent. Interestingly, no change was noted in the percentage of people who did not discuss CAM use with their physicians: Approximately 60 percent did not discuss CAM use with their physicians in both studies.

Several U.S. studies indicate that the use of CAM continues to be relatively high and will be high in the future. A large analysis of CAM use in the U.S. was conducted in 2002 (3). In this survey, 50 percent of the general population had, at one time or another, used some form of CAM (excluding two widely used therapies, prayer and exercise). Another U.S. study found that CAM use is not a short-lived fad (4). In this report, CAM use by the age of 33 was evaluated relative to birth date. For those born before 1945, about 30 percent of respondents used CAM. The percentage of CAM users rose to about 50 percent for those born between 1945 and 1964, and was even higher, about 70 percent, for those born between 1965 and 1979. This study also found that nearly one-half of people who tried a specific form of CAM continued to use that CAM therapy more than 20 years later. Overall, this study indicates that CAM is not a short-lived phenomenon because some CAM therapies are used long-term and CAM use in general is higher among younger people.

Several studies of the general population have identified certain characteristics of CAM users. CAM use tends to be higher in women and in those who have conditions that lack definitive cures, have unpredictable courses, and are associated with discomfort, pain, and side effects from prescription medications. Because these are characteristics of MS and people with MS, these findings suggest that CAM use may be more prevalent in people with MS than in the general population.

CAM Use in MS

Several studies have evaluated CAM use in MS. One of the earliest studies was conducted in Massachusetts and California in the 1990s (5). Approximately 60 percent of people had used CAM, and, on average, people used two to three different types of CAM. We conducted a similar survey, in 1997, at the Rocky Mountain Multiple Sclerosis Center and found that approximately two-thirds of those who responded to the survey used CAM.

Several subsequent studies have investigated CAM use in people with MS. If one evaluates the results of various U.S. studies of CAM use among people with MS, and if one uses a definition of CAM that includes therapies that have ever been used and excludes two widely used therapies (prayer and exercise), 50 to 88 percent of people with MS have used CAM (5–9). As noted previously, a 2002 study of the general population in the U.S., using a similar definition of CAM, found that 50 percent of people use CAM. It is difficult to compare studies with such different methodologies. However, rough comparisons of these various studies indicate that the use of CAM in people with MS appears to be similar to or somewhat higher than that in the general population.

A different type of study, reported in 1999, examined visits to CAM practitioners by people with MS (10). This study did not evaluate overall CAM use and, of note, most people who use CAM do not visit a practitioner. CAM practitioner use in this study, which was about one-third, was higher than the rate of about 10 percent reported for CAM practitioner use in several studies of the general population done during the 1990s.

The use of CAM among people with MS does not appear to be an American phenomenon. Studies of other countries indicate similar results for the percentage of people with MS who use CAM: 82.5 percent in Australia, 70 percent in Canada, 27 to 55 percent in Denmark, and 41 percent in Spain (11–14).

In surveys of people with MS and of the general population, a consistent finding is that CAM usually is used in conjunction with conventional medical therapy. In other words, CAM usually is used in a complementary way. Approximately 90 percent of people who use CAM also use conventional medicine. This leaves a relatively small fraction of people who use CAM in a truly alternative manner.

It is sometimes erroneously believed that only two preference groups for medical therapy exist: one group that uses only conventional therapy and another group that uses only CAM therapy. In fact, a third "mixed" group combines conventional medicine and CAM. Of importance, the studies of CAM use in people with MS demonstrate not only that this "mixed" group exists but also that it actually appears to represent the majority of people with MS.

With a large number of people with MS pursuing CAM therapies, it is essential for people to be knowledgeable about the therapies they choose and for physicians, other health care providers, and CAM practitioners to be aware that multiple conventional and CAM therapies are in use and that interactions among them are possible.

People with MS use a wide range of CAM therapies. Those that appear to be especially popular include massage, dietary supplements, diets, chiropractic medicine, acupuncture, meditation and guided imagery, and yoga.

The reasons why people with MS pursue CAM are as varied as the different CAM modalities used. "Curing MS" is not a frequently cited reason for using CAM. Common reasons include decreasing the severity of MS-associated symptoms, increasing control, improving health, and using a method that accounts for the interrelation of mind, body, and spirit. Some people are drawn to CAM because of the lack of effectiveness of conventional medications and anecdotal reports of benefits or recommendations from friends, relatives, or physicians (5,8,12). One study of CAM use in people with MS and other chronic diseases concluded that CAM was an important component for self-care and was not generally embraced as a rejection of conventional medicine or an unrealistic search for a cure (15).

Some characteristics have been reported more frequently in those with MS who use CAM. These include being female, having a lower level of health, and being more highly educated. One recent study also found that people who used CAM were less likely to use one of the FDA-approved MS medications and were more likely to have a lower level of physical well-being (9).

Information About CAM and MS

For CAM in general, the information available to the general public is vast but of variable quality. For CAM that is relevant to MS, the amount of information is limited and the quality also is variable. To attempt to understand the type of information that is available on CAM and MS, we conducted an informal survey of the popular literature on CAM at the Rocky Mountain Multiple Sclerosis Center. At two local bookstores, we found 50 CAM books written for a lay audience. Two-thirds of these books had sections on MS. In some books, MS was incorrectly defined as a form of muscular dystrophy. Other books made the erroneous—and potentially dangerous—statement that, because MS is an immune disorder, it is important to take supplements that stimulate the immune system. In fact, MS is an immune disorder, but it is characterized by an excessively active immune system; thus, immune-stimulating supplements actually may be harmful. On average, the CAM books recommended five or six therapies for MS. In 20 percent of them, 10 or more therapies were recommended. It was rare for books to discourage the use of any CAM treatment. Interestingly, none had the same recommended therapies. In general, therapies that are used more frequently by patients appear to be those that are recommended more often in books; the fact that this information contains inaccuracies is therefore troubling.

In addition to books, information about CAM can be obtained from vendors of products and CAM practitioners. Unfortunately, product vendors, such as people who sell supplements, often exaggerate claims about their products. Practitioners of CAM (as well as product vendors) sometimes have limited experience with MS and are not certain how their therapy relates to such a specific and complex disease process.

Physicians and other mainstream health care providers are another potential source of information about CAM. Unfortunately, this group generally is not trained or experienced in CAM use and, for a variety of reasons, often is reluctant to become involved in this area. Even for conventional health care providers who are interested in CAM, only a limited amount of objective and accessible MS-specific information is currently available in the medical literature.

People with MS are "Caught in the Middle"

Many people with MS pursue some form of CAM but may not readily be able to obtain objective and practical information. They may seek out CAM books, products, or practitioners, but find that MS is not specifically addressed or that claims of the effectiveness of the therapy are exaggerated. On the other hand, they may attempt to obtain CAM information from their physician or other health care provider and find that little or no information is available. In this way, pursuing CAM can be frustrating and confusing for people with MS.

A Website Focused on CAM and MS

This book was written to provide objective, MS-relevant CAM information to people with MS. Also, because the area of CAM is changing rapidly, we developed a website devoted to CAM and MS at the Rocky Mountain Multiple Sclerosis Center. This site, www.ms-cam.org, is updated regularly and has interactive features. This site has several missions:

- To create a worldwide community of people interested in CAM and MS
- To provide accurate and unbiased information
- To allow users to discuss their experiences with CAM through threaded discussions
- To conduct surveys to assess the effectiveness and safety of CAM therapies for people with MS

A Matter of Perspective

CAM is controversial for many different reasons. One important issue to keep in mind is that of *perspective*. Because of differences in perspective, mainstream health care providers and people with a disease may view the same set of facts differently.

Physicians view the use of basic science and rigorous clinical trial methods as a powerful tool to develop new disease understanding and new therapies. People with MS may believe that this process is powerful, but that it is also slow and may yield limited advances during their lifetimes.

The "gold standard" for developing new therapies is a randomized, controlled clinical trial. This clinical testing employs specific and rigorous methods, including the use of a placebo-treated group, "blinding" of patients and investigators (so that neither patients nor investigators know who has received placebo and who has received active medication), and randomly selecting those who will receive placebo or active medication. Physicians and other mainstream health care providers generally use therapies only after they have been found to be effective in these well-designed clinical trials. Through this process, a black-and-white distinction exists between those therapies that have been proven effective in clinical trials and those that have not.

Some of the interest in and controversy over CAM stems from the fact that there may not be such a black-and-white distinction, but rather shades of gray. For example, some therapies have not undergone rigorous large-scale clinical testing, but scientific studies in animals or small clinical studies in people have produced promising results. These types of therapies generally are not incorporated into mainstream medicine. However, people with a disease may have an interest in such promising therapies, especially if they are relatively safe and inexpensive.

Another difference in patient–physician perspective is apparent with proven mainstream therapies. Conventional medications that are 30 to 40 percent effective may represent a major advance for physicians and other health care providers but, for people with MS, these therapies may be seen as 60 to 70 percent away from a cure (which would be 100 percent effective).

In some areas of CAM, the same set of facts is viewed negatively by conventional medicine and positively by some people with MS. This emphasizes the importance of first establishing the facts about a therapy and then realizing that these facts may be interpreted differently by mainstream health care providers and people with MS. Under some circumstances, it is as if two different cultures exist: that of the health care provider and that of the person who has the disease. These two cultures may have strikingly different belief systems.

The difference in perspective becomes especially apparent when a physician develops a disease. In this situation, a dramatic shift may occur in an individual's attitudes about what constitutes an appropriate medical therapy. There have been several published examples of this shift in perspective.

Dr. Alexander Burnfield, an English psychiatrist who has MS, wrote a book entitled *Multiple Sclerosis: A Personal Exploration*. With reference to evening primrose oil, he states: "I started taking it before the research was published and, being only human, take it just in case I get worse if I stop. This is, I know, an unscientific and emotional response, and the logical-doctor part of me is quite shocked" (16).

Dr. Elizabeth Forsythe, also an English physician with MS, wrote *Multiple Sclerosis: Exploring Sickness and Health*. With reference to diet and MS, she states: "It is what you feel in your own body and mind that is the most important thing, and it is very easy for doctors and patients to forget that. I believe that a little of what you fancy does do you good!" (17).

In *Healing Lessons*, Dr. Sidney Winawer, chief of gastroenterology at Memorial–Sloan Kettering Hospital in New York City, gives a provocative account of his transformational experiences with CAM through his relationship with his wife, who pursues various unconventional and unproven cancer therapies. He writes: "I failed to see that Andrea's cancer, of all things, would wake us up. I knew least of all that my beliefs as a doctor were about to be turned upside down" (18). He also begins to view therapies from a different perspective: "I shared her conviction that uncertain hope was better than hopeless certainty" (19).

A Unified Perspective

Should we abandon these mainstream methods because basic science research has not fully elucidated the cause of MS and clinical trials have not developed a cure? NO. These methods of conventional medicine provide the greatest hope for understanding and curing MS. The difficulty is that MS is a complex disease, and an uncertain amount of future work is needed.

Should we acknowledge that areas of CAM exist that may be of interest to people with MS because conventional medicine does not have a cure for MS? YES. It is a disservice to people with MS who have an interest in CAM to not acknowledge that these therapies exist. Part of this acknowledgment should involve providing accurate information. By focusing more attention on CAM, we may actually develop a new understanding of the disease process and perhaps discover new therapies.

It is possible to simultaneously acknowledge, respect, and use conventional medical therapy and CAM therapy. This dual approach is a way to bring together the sometimes disparate views of mainstream health care providers and people with MS.

Additional Readings

Websites

www.ms-cam.org. CAM website of the Rocky Mountain Multiple Sclerosis Center

Books

Bourdette D, Yadav V, Shinto L. Multiple sclerosis. In: Oken BS, ed. *Complementary Therapies in Neurology: An Evidence-Based Approach.* New York: Parthenon Publishing Group, 2004, 291–302.

Burnfield A. *Multiple Sclerosis: A Personal Exploration.* London: Souvenir Press, 1997.

Cassileth BR. *The Alternative Medicine Handbook.* New York: W.W. Norton, 1998.

Ernst E, ed. *The Desktop Guide to Complementary and Alternative Medicine: An Evidence-Based Approach.* Edinburgh: Mosby, 2001.

Forsythe E. *Multiple Sclerosis: Exploring Sickness and Health.* London: Faber and Faber, 1988.

Freeman L. *Mosby's Complementary and Alternative Medicine: A Research-Based Approach.* St. Louis: Mosby, 2004.

Institute of Medicine. Committee on the Use of Complementary and Alternative Medicine by the American Public. *Complementary and Alternative Medicine in the United States.* Washington, D.C.: National Academies Press, 2005.

Kalb RC. *Multiple Sclerosis: The Questions You Have—The Answers You Need.* New York: Demos Medical Publishing, 2004.

Navarra T. *The Encyclopedia of Complementary and Alternative Medicine.* New York: Checkmark Books, 2005.

Polman CH, Thompson AJ, Murray TJ, et al. *Multiple Sclerosis: The Guide to Treatment and Management.* New York: Demos Medical Publishing, 2006.

Schapiro RT. *Managing the Symptoms of Multiple Sclerosis.* New York: Demos Medical Publishing, 2003.

Spencer JW, Jacobs JJ. *Complementary/Alternative Medicine: An Evidence-Based Approach.* St. Louis: Mosby, 2003.

Winawer SJ. *Healing Lessons.* Boston: Little, Brown, 1998.

Journal Articles

Barnes PM, Powell-Griner E, McFann K, et al. Complementary and alternative medicine use among adults: United States, 2002. *Adv Data* 2004;343:1–20.

Berkman CS, Pignotti MG, Cavallo PF, et al. Use of alternative treatments by people with multiple sclerosis. *Neurorehab Neural Repair* 1999;13:243–254.

Bowling AC. Complementary and alternative medicine in multiple sclerosis: dispelling common myths about CAM. *Int J MS Care* 2005;7:42–44.

Bowling AC, Ibrahim R, Stewart TM. Alternative medicine and multiple sclerosis: an objective review from an American perspective. *Int J MS Care* 2000;2:14–21.

Bowling AC, Stewart TM. Current complementary and alternative therapies of multiple sclerosis. *Curr Treatment Options Neurol* 2003;5:55–68.

Eisenberg D, Davis R, Ettner S, et al. Trends in alternative medicine use in the United States, 1990–1997. *JAMA* 1998;280:1569–1575.

Eisenberg D, Kessler R, Foster C, et al. Unconventional medicine in the United States. *N Engl J Med* 1993;328:246–252.

Schwartz C, Laitin E, Brotman S, et al. Utilization of unconventional treatments by persons with MS: is it alternative or complementary? *Neurology* 1999;52:626–629.

Shinto L, Yadav V, Morris C, et al. Demographic and health-related factors associated with complementary and alternative medicine (CAM) use in multiple sclerosis. *Mult Scler* 2006;12:94–100.

Tindle HA, Davis RB, Phillips RS, et al. Trends in use of complementary and alternative medicine by US adults: 1997–2002. *Alt Ther* 2005;11:42–49.

2

Placebos and Psychoneuroimmunology

When considering any type of medicine, whether unconventional or conventional, it is important to understand and recognize the significance of placebos and the placebo effect. The beneficial effects of placebos highlight the complexity of treating human disease and are necessary to consider when evaluating the effects of any therapy.

Placebos and the Placebo Effect

A placebo is generally thought of as a "dummy pill" or "sugar pill." More formally, a placebo is a therapy that is not believed to have a specific effect on the disease or the condition for which it is given. *Placebo* is derived from Latin and means, "I will please." A placebo may be given in the form of a substance or a procedure. The *placebo effect* is the response of a person's condition to the placebo.

Many dramatic examples of the placebo effect exist. One of the early examples in medical literature involved a woman with excessive nausea and vomiting during pregnancy. She was told she was being given a medication for nausea but was actually given syrup of ipecac, which is known to induce vomiting and is sometimes given to children who have swallowed a possibly toxic substance. The woman in this study actually had improvement in her nausea.

A well-known study of the placebo effect was reported in 1955 by Dr. Harry Beecher (1). He described the placebo effect in a variety of conditions, including the common cold, pain after surgery, headache, and seasickness. Overall, symptoms were improved in 35 percent of the people who were given the placebo. Subsequent studies of a variety of medical conditions found placebo effects that were frequently in the range of 30 to 40 percent. In some studies, placebos have been 70 percent effective.

As would be expected, a placebo effect occurs in studies of people with multiple sclerosis (MS). A notable response to placebos has been observed in studies of therapy for MS itself, as well as for MS-related symptoms. In older MS studies, from 1935 to 1950, a variety of ineffective therapies produced 60 to 70 percent improvement. More recently, trials with chemotherapy drugs in MS showed a placebo effect on the rate of MS attacks. In recent research studies using interferon beta-1b (Betaseron), the first U.S. Food and Drug Administration (FDA)-approved immune therapy for MS, the number of MS attacks was determined for people taking Betaseron and for another group taking placebo. The placebo-treated group had a 28 percent decrease in the rate of MS attacks. Similarly, the placebo group showed decreased attack rates of 33 percent in trials using intramuscular interferon beta-1a (Avonex), 13 percent in trials with subcutaneous interferon beta-1a (Rebif), and 43 percent in trials with glatiramer acetate (Copaxone). In all these trials, the study drug was significantly more effective than the placebo, and this finding is the basis for the widespread use of these medications.

Several explanations can be given for the decrease in MS attack rates observed with placebos. This may represent the natural course of the disease, or it may be an artifact of statistics (referred to as *regression to the mean*), but it also may represent a genuine placebo effect.

Placebo responses also have occurred in studies that use biologic tests to monitor disease activity. Magnetic resonance imaging (MRI) is frequently used in MS clinical trials. A recent MRI study of a small number of people with MS found that the placebo-treated group had an approximately 20 percent reduction in the development of new brain lesions (2). This finding was not statistically significant, but this may have been due to the small number of people in the study.

A particularly interesting finding occurred in a study of an experimental medication, alpha-interferon (3). People with MS were given alpha-interferon or placebo. They were evaluated by determining the rate of attacks. Both the treated group and the placebo group had a 60 to 70 percent decline in the rate of MS attacks. The investigators also measured the activity of an immune cell known as a *natural killer cell*. The natural killer cell activity was evaluated because it is known that its activity is increased by alpha-interferon. As expected, the group treated with alpha-interferon showed a 52 percent increase in natural killer cell activity. Surprisingly, the placebo group showed an increase in natural killer cell activity that was nearly identical to that of the alpha-interferon group.

Placebo effects have been observed in other MS clinical studies, including those that have evaluated treatment for symptoms caused by the disease. For MS-associated fatigue, the placebo effect in clinical trials has been as high as 50 percent.

These studies suggest that the mind may have a powerful influence over a disease process such as MS, as well as over the activity of the immune system.

Interaction of the Nervous System and the Immune System

In the past, little interaction was thought to occur between the nervous system and the immune system. However, recent studies demonstrate that there *are* ways in which the nervous system and the immune system communicate with each other. The placebo effects observed in people with MS and other diseases may be examples of this process. The field of study that examines immune system–nervous system interactions has been termed *psychoneuroimmunology*.

The brain may communicate with the immune system in many different ways. The brain influences the production of hormones, which then may affect the function of the immune system. In addition, nerve fibers have connections with immune organs. The chemical messengers used by the nervous and immune systems appear to be involved in cross-communication. Nerve cells communicate with each other by releasing chemicals known as neurotransmitters, whereas immune cells communicate with each other by secreting different chemicals, known as *cytokines*. Research studies have shown that cytokines may influence nerve-cell activity and that neurotransmitters may influence immune-cell function. Thus, the nervous system and the immune system do not appear to function independently but rather are components of a network in which they communicate and alter each others' activity.

Because there appear to be important interactions between the nervous system and the immune system, modifying brain activity may alter the immune system and immune diseases such as MS. For example, psychological stress and depression may influence the functioning of the immune system. One way to manage stress is to write about stressful life events. The act of writing about such events has been associated with improved immune function and improvement in two immune diseases, rheumatoid arthritis and asthma.

A variety of studies have evaluated the influence of the nervous system on MS activity. In animals, injury to one component of the peripheral nerves (nerves that are outside the brain and spinal cord)—the sympathetic nervous system—leads to altered immune function and worsening of experimental allergic encephalomyelitis (EAE), an animal model of MS.

Many studies have examined the possible influence of psychological stress on MS. In this area, two large questions exist. The first question is: Does stress cause MS attacks? For the first question, several individual studies (4) and a combined analysis of these studies (5), known as a meta-analysis, indicate that the risk of attacks increases after stressful life events. At this time, however, this is still a "chicken-or-the-egg" question. That is, it is possible that stress actually causes attacks. Alternatively, the earliest manifestation of an attack could be stress, in which case the attack causes stress. Interestingly, in the meta-analysis, the magnitude of the negative effect of stress (53 percent) was similar to the magnitude of the positive effect of the injectable MS medications (36 percent).

Another question in this area is whether stress worsens chronic MS symptoms. For example, if someone with MS has muscle stiffness on a daily basis, can times of increased stress be associated with increased stiffness? Limited studies in this area indicate that stress may indeed increase the severity of chronic symptoms.

Placebos and CAM

Placebos and the placebo effect are important when considering conventional and unconventional medicine. In conventional medicine, the placebo effect often is disregarded or minimized. In clinical trials of experimental drugs, the placebo response is simply subtracted from the effect of the drug. Also, a certain level of discomfort exists for placebos within conventional medicine. Dr. Jay Katz states: "… if placebos were to be acknowledged as effective in their own right, it would expose large gaps in medicine's and in doctors' knowledge about underlying mechanisms of care and relief from suffering" (6).

For studies of MS, which is an extremely individualized, variable, and unpredictable disease, it is clear that any evaluated therapy must be compared with a placebo. Sometimes CAM therapies are touted on the basis of the experience of individuals; these are known as *anecdotes*. Because of the placebo effect and the fact that MS may remain stable with no therapy or that full recovery may occur after an MS attack, it is important not to rely heavily on treatment benefits based only on anecdotes. Whether a therapy is conventional or unconventional, definitive claims of effectiveness must be based on studies of large numbers of people, some of whom are treated with placebos.

Finally, an important difference between conventional medicine and CAM may relate to the placebo effect. It has been stated that much of the history of medicine is actually the history of the placebo effect because medicine has not, until recently, had particularly effective therapies. Physicians in the past may have relied very heavily on establishing relationships with patients and may have become skilled at administering ineffective therapies in a way that maximized the placebo response.

Modern mainstream medicine has undergone significant changes. It has become more technological. Much of medicine is now focused on the body alone, instead of on the body and the mind. Decreased insurance reimbursement has led to briefer physician visits. With all these changes, many physicians lack the resources and time to nurture strong patient relationships and to develop optimal methods for administering therapies. In contrast to the past history of medicine, the recent history of some aspects of American medicine may be the history of removing the placebo effect from clinical practice.

In contrast to physicians, many practitioners of CAM probably spend more time with patients and rely more on positive interpersonal skills to interact with and treat them. This may be true for practitioners in areas such as acupuncture, homeopathy, and massage. A single session with these practitioners may last 60 minutes or longer and involve a detailed discussion of many topics, whereas physician visits are often 10 to 20 minutes or shorter and focus exclusively on diseases, symptoms, diagnostic tests, and drug therapies. Regardless of the effectiveness of their therapies, some practitioners of CAM may be more skilled and more comfortable than are physicians with using the power of the placebo effect.

Additional Readings

Books

Brody H. *The Placebo Response*. New York: HarperCollins, 2000.

Evans D. *Placebo: The Belief Effect*. London: HarperCollins, 2003.

Harrington A, ed. *The Placebo Effect: An Interdisciplinary Exploration*. Cambridge: Harvard University Press, 1997.

Moerman D. *Meaning, Medicine, and the Placebo Effect*. Cambridge: Cambridge University Press, 2002.

Oken B. Placebo effect: clinical perspectives and potential mechanisms. In: Oken BS, ed. *Complementary Therapies In Neurology: An Evidence-Based Approach*. New York: Parthenon Publishing Group, 2004, 209–230.

Shapiro AK, Shapiro E. *The Powerful Placebo*. Baltimore: Johns Hopkins University Press, 1997.

Journal Articles

Benedetti F. Recent advances in placebo research. *Int J Pain Med Pall Care* 2005;4:2–7.

Brown RF, Tennant CC, Dunn SM, et al. A review of stress-relapse interactions in multiple sclerosis: important features and stress-mediating and -moderating variables. *Mult Scler* 2005;11:477–484.

Chelmicka-Schorr E, Arnason BG. Nervous system–immune system interactions and their role in multiple sclerosis. *Ann Neurol* 1994;36:S29–S32.

Hirsch RL, Johnson KP, Camenga DL. The placebo effect during a double blind trial of recombinant alpha2 interferon in multiple sclerosis patients: immunological and clinical findings. *Neuroscience* 1988;39:189–196.

La Mantia L, Eoli M, Salmaggi A, et al. Does a placebo-effect exist in clinical trials on multiple sclerosis? Review of the literature. *Ital J Neurol Sci* 1996;17:135–139.

3

Important Precautions About Complementary and Alternative Medicine and MS

This book provides much detailed information about specific types of complementary and alternative medicine (CAM). This information is intended to assist people in assessing CAM therapies for multiple sclerosis (MS). In addition to this specific information, some general ideas are important to understand and may be helpful in the CAM decision-making process:

- *The information in this book should not be used to "convert" anyone to CAM therapy use, and it should not be taken as a recommendation to use specific types of CAM.* Conclusive evidence about the effectiveness and safety of most forms of CAM is not available. Consequently, this book provides information but does not make recommendations. Because this book does not specifically promote the use of CAM, individuals who are not interested in CAM should not feel any need for "conversion" to it. For those individuals who already are interested in CAM, the information in this book should be helpful in assessing the possible effectiveness, safety, and cost of different therapies. Without specific recommendations, the way in which the information is used and the decision about whether to pursue CAM therapy rests with the individual. Ultimately, individuals must decide for themselves about using CAM, and they must assume the risks and responsibilities of pursuing a specific CAM therapy.

- *Be aware of when it is reasonable to pursue CAM.* It is reasonable to consider CAM therapy in some situations. For example, it would be reasonable to consider CAM for a symptom that is of low intensity, such as mild muscle stiffness or mild pain. CAM also may be worth pursuing for a condition in which conventional medical therapy is ineffective or only partially effective. Forms of CAM to consider are those that are possibly effective, are probably safe, are of low or moderate cost, and require only a reasonable amount of effort. On the other hand, severe symptoms, such as prominent muscle stiffness or excruciating pain, or a serious disease process—such as MS—should not be treated *solely* with CAM. In these situations, it may be reasonable to pursue CAM *in addition to* conventional therapy. In other words, using CAM in a complementary way may be appropriate. CAM therapy should not be pursued if little or no reliable information is available about effectiveness, safety, or cost. Therapies to avoid are those that are probably ineffective or unsafe or involve high expense or great effort.

■ *Have a plan for using CAM.* Several steps must be taken when using any form of CAM:

   ■ Consider conventional medicine first
   ■ Evaluate and address the reason(s) for wanting to use CAM
   ■ Obtain accurate information about effectiveness, safety, cost, and effort involved
   ■ If CAM is chosen, discuss it with your physician, monitor your response, and discontinue the treatment when appropriate
   ■ Use caution

It is important to include a physician in this process because most CAM practitioners do not have a physician's broad knowledge base about the diagnosis and treatment of medical conditions.

■ *Realize that information about most forms of CAM is incomplete.* Many forms of conventional medical therapy have undergone rigorous testing for effectiveness and safety. In contrast, data are limited for most CAM therapies, especially in terms of specialized studies of people with MS or studies of the effects of therapies on immune-system activity. As a result, often it is only possible to make a "best guess" about the effectiveness and safety of CAM. As more studies are done on CAM, some of these "best guesses" may be found to be incorrect. For example, a therapy that is currently thought to be "possibly effective" or "probably safe" may conceivably be found, after further studies, to be definitely ineffective or definitely unsafe. Thus, a certain amount of risk is involved in pursuing CAM. In terms of slowing down the MS disease process, no "magic cure" exists. No forms of CAM therapy have undergone sophisticated clinical testing similar to that used to prove the efficacy of glatiramer acetate (Copaxone), interferon beta-1b (Betaseron), interferon beta-1a (Avonex and Rebif), mitoxantrone (Novantrone), and natalizumab (Tysabri). As a result, these therapies should be considered by all people with MS before pursuing CAM.

■　*Be aware of the "telltale signs" of unreliable forms of CAM.* Several features often indicate that a CAM therapy has not been well studied, is provided by an unreliable source, or is being promoted with exaggerated claims. Some of these "telltale signs" are:

- ■　Heavy reliance on testimonials: The benefits of a therapy sometimes are reported in accounts known as *testimonials*, which may not be entirely accurate and which describe the treatment response of a single person, as opposed to that of a large, well-studied group of people.
- ■　Strong claims about effectiveness: Terms such as "amazing" and "miraculous" should raise suspicions. If it sounds too good to be true, it probably is.
- ■　A single therapy is claimed to be effective for many different medical conditions.
- ■　The composition of a therapy is "secret."
- ■　Little or no objective information is available on effectiveness, safety, or cost.
- ■　Therapy involves inpatient treatment, injections, or intravenous medication.
- ■　An antiscience or anticonventional medicine attitude prevails: This may be conveyed through claims of "conspiracies" or through the unwillingness of a CAM practitioner to work cooperatively with a physician.

■　*Recognize that MS is a disease that involves excessive immune system activity.* In some lay books on CAM, MS is described as an immune disorder, and it is then assumed that therapies that stimulate the immune system should be beneficial for MS. Some books may even recommend 5 to 10 supplements that activate the immune system. Using this faulty reasoning, therapies recommended for MS are sometimes the same as those recommended for acquired immunodeficiency syndrome (AIDS) and cancer. Also, the vague term *immunomodulator* sometimes is used to describe supplements that appear to stimulate the immune system. This approach and these recommendations are inaccurate and potentially dangerous. Although MS is, indeed, an immune disorder, it generally involves too much, not too little, immune-system activity. Consequently, CAM therapies that increase the activity of the immune system could worsen the disease process. In contrast to MS, AIDS and cancer may benefit from treatment that activates the immune system. Thus, in general, immune-stimulating therapies that may be helpful for AIDS and cancer may actually be harmful for MS.

■ *Do not confuse scientific evidence with clinical evidence.* Potential MS therapies may be evaluated scientifically through "test tube" experiments or by using an animal model of MS known as experimental allergic encephalomyelitis (EAE). The most important (and most expensive and laborious) test of a therapy, however, is to give it to people with MS and to carefully monitor their response. It is essential to realize that scientific studies are imperfect and that therapies that are promising in scientific experiments are not necessarily clinically effective therapies for people with MS. A long list of experimental compounds are effective in suppressing the immune system or treating EAE but are ineffective for treating people with MS. Some therapies (for example, interferon-gamma, lenercept, and antibodies to tumor necrosis factor [TNF]) are effective in treating animal models of MS but actually worsen disease in people with MS.

■ *Avoid misconceptions about supplements.* Many misconceptions are sometimes promoted by the vendors of supplements. These misconceptions include:

■ Compounds are sometimes claimed to be safe and beneficial if they are "natural." Although some natural compounds are safe and beneficial, some are toxic (for example, the deadly chemicals that are present in poisonous mushrooms and many other plants), and many are not effective therapies for any disorder.

■ Some supplements, especially herbs, are claimed to have beneficial effects and no side effects. Supplements (like prescription medications) that have beneficial effects must contain chemicals that also may potentially produce side effects.

■ *More is not necessarily better.* It is sometimes believed that the use of high doses of a single supplement or a large number of different supplements is more beneficial than the use of low doses or a single supplement; however, in most cases, supplements in high doses or large numbers are probably not more effective and may, in fact, be more likely to produce side effects.

■ *Combinations of supplements with conventional medications have not been fully investigated.* Supplements are sometimes taken in addition to conventional medications (for example, evening primrose oil and one of the FDA-approved injectable MS medications); the effectiveness and safety of these "combination therapies" has not been investigated. Notably, some situations exist in which combination therapy is less effective or more likely to produce side effects than single-treatment therapy.

The precautions discussed in this introduction have been incorporated into the discussions in this book. These guidelines should be helpful for evaluating CAM therapies not mentioned here or for assessing CAM therapies for conditions other than MS.

Types of Therapy

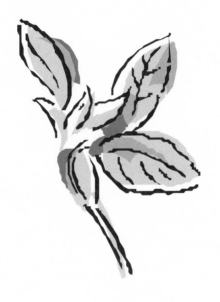

4

Acupuncture and Traditional Chinese Medicine

*A*cupuncture is one of many components of what is known as traditional Chinese medicine, a healing method that has been in use for more than 2,000 years. Traditional Chinese medicine is used by approximately one-fourth of the world's population. In Western countries, the use of traditional Chinese medicine, especially acupuncture, has grown over the past two decades. It is estimated that more than one million Americans are treated with acupuncture yearly.

The recognition of acupuncture by Western medicine is not entirely new. In the late 1800s, Sir William Osler, one of the most honored and respected physicians and medical educators, wrote a textbook of medicine in which he recommended acupuncture for low back pain and sciatica. In 1901, *Gray's Anatomy*, a classic medical text, also referred to acupuncture as a treatment for sciatica.

There are five components of traditional Chinese medicine. In addition to acupuncture, they include traditional Chinese herbs, diet and nutrition, exercise, stress reduction and counseling, and massage. T'ai chi, which is discussed elsewhere in this book, is also a component of traditional Chinese medicine. This chapter discusses acupuncture as well as two types of herbal medicine: Asian herbal medicine and Asian proprietary (or patent) medicine.

Acupuncture

Acupuncture is based on a complex theory of body functioning that is very different from the Western biologic approach. Briefly, it is believed that a free flow of energy or *qi* passes through 12 major pathways or *meridians* on the body. A balance of opposites also exists, known as *yin* and *yang*. Disease is believed to result from a disruption in the normal flow of this energy.

Treatment Method

Acupuncture involves the insertion of thin, solid, metallic needles into specific points on the meridians. It is believed that this alters the flow of energy and thereby produces improvement. Approximately 400 acupuncture points exist. Fortunately, not all these are used in a single session! Four to 12 points are typically used in a session.

For those wary of needles, methods other than needle insertion may be used to stimulate acupuncture points. The application of finger pressure to these points is known as *acupressure* or, in Japan, *shiatsu*. Small hot cups are placed on points with *cupping*, and electrically stimulated needles are used with *electroacupuncture*. Transcutaneous electrical nerve stimulation (TENS), a variant of electroacupuncture, sometimes is used. In *moxibustion*, smoldering fibers of an herb, Asian mugwort or "moxa," are placed on acupuncture points or are used to heat needles that are then placed in acupuncture points.

How could a needle stuck into the skin possibly provide pain relief and other medical benefits? Many answers to this question have been proposed. As noted, from a traditional Chinese medicine perspective, the insertion of needles is believed to alter the flow of energy in such a way that it produces therapeutic effects. From a Western scientific viewpoint, various possible mechanisms have been explored. One explanation for the pain-relieving effects of acupuncture is that it releases *opioids*, chemicals produced by the body that decrease pain. Other studies indicate that levels of another chemical, *serotonin*, are altered by acupuncture. Studies on the brain using magnetic resonance imaging (MRI) indicate that acupuncture may change the activity in specific pain-related brain regions. Acupuncture also may decrease stress or, in some situations, act as a placebo. In the end, it may be found that multiple processes are involved.

Studies in MS and Other Conditions

A large number of studies have evaluated the effectiveness of acupuncture. Unfortunately, many of these studies have been small and not well conducted. To attempt to understand the possible medical benefits of acupuncture, the National Institutes of Health (NIH) organized a 12-member panel in 1997 to review the studies on acupuncture (1). The panel concluded that there existed "clear evidence" for acupuncture's effectiveness in relieving nausea and vomiting associated with surgery, chemotherapy, and possibly pregnancy. Evidence for effectiveness also was found for pain after dental procedures and several other types of pain. The report concluded that "the data in support of acupuncture are as strong as those for many accepted Western medical therapies" and that acupuncture was a "reasonable option" for some conditions.

It is surprising how few studies have evaluated acupuncture in multiple sclerosis (MS). In 1974, a Canadian study of eight people with MS showed that a few had some mild and brief benefits (2). However, there did not appear to be long-lasting effects. In 1986, a very small study of two people with MS showed that multiple MS symptoms improved (3). A recent preliminary study indicates that acupuncture may improve MS-related bladder difficulties.

Interesting and contrary results have been obtained in small studies of the effects of acupuncture on MS-associated muscle stiffness, which is also known as *spasticity*. One study evaluated four people with MS—two of these people were wheelchair-bound and the other two were able to walk (4). Improvement in spasticity was seen in the two people who were able to walk but not in those who were wheelchair-bound. A 1986 study of 28 people with MS evaluated responses to stimulation at acupuncture sites (5). Interestingly, acupuncture sites were more sensitive in people with MS, and needle insertion provoked stiffness and muscle spasms. These findings may simply reflect a generalized MS-associated skin hypersensitivity or vulnerability to muscle stiffness.

Two large surveys have evaluated the effects of acupuncture on people with MS. At the Rocky Mountain Multiple Sclerosis Center, we conducted a web-based survey on acupuncture on our CAM website, www.ms-cam.org. The preliminary results have been reported (6) and may be viewed at the website. Among more than 1,000 respondents, about 20 percent had used acupuncture since they were diagnosed with MS. The symptoms that were reported to be improved most frequently were pain and anxiety—about two-thirds reported improvement with these symptoms. Other symptoms that were reported by 50 to 60 percent of people to be improved were fatigue, depression, muscle stiffness, numbness, and insomnia. Acupuncture was reported to be well-tolerated generally. About 4 percent noted worsening of a pre-existing MS symptom with acupuncture. About 4 percent also noted that acupuncture caused a new symptom—the most common new symptoms were dizziness, pain, and decreased balance.

Another survey evaluated acupuncture use in 217 people with MS in British Columbia (7). The preliminary results of this survey indicate that approximately two-thirds reported beneficial effects. Many symptoms were improved, including pain, spasticity, bowel and bladder difficulties, tingling, weakness, walking difficulties, incoordination, and sleep disorders. The few side effects that were reported were pain and soreness at the needle site and a worsening of some symptoms (fatigue, spasticity, dizziness, and walking unsteadiness).

Overall, the results of these surveys are promising. However, it must be kept in mind that these are self-assessment surveys, not formal clinical trials.

Some studies have evaluated the effectiveness of acupuncture for symptoms that may occur with MS. In these studies, however, the underlying disease was not MS. Limited studies suggest beneficial effects of acupuncture for weakness in people with strokes. In studies of variable quality, it has been found that acupuncture may be effective for other symptoms that may occur with MS, including anxiety, depression, pain (including headache, facial pain, low back pain, and neck pain), dizziness, sleeping difficulties, and urinary difficulties.

An important issue for MS is whether acupuncture has an effect on the immune system. At this time, the impact of acupuncture on immune-system activity is not well understood. Although no studies have been done specifically in people with MS, acupuncture studies on immune-system activity have been done in people with various forms of cancer and rheumatoid arthritis. Acupuncture has been associated with stimulating, inhibiting, and having no effect on the immune system. Because of these mixed results, further studies are needed to clarify this area.

Given the probable benefits of acupuncture in other medical conditions, it would be reasonable to pursue detailed studies of its effects in MS. Rigorous studies of the effect of acupuncture on the course of the disease would be expensive and difficult. In contrast, it would be feasible to evaluate the effects of acupuncture on some MS-associated symptoms, including pain, spasticity, weakness, and urinary disorders. If acupuncture were found to be effective for symptoms, it could be a useful therapy. However, the treatment of chronic symptoms might need to be long-term, which may not be practical.

Side Effects

In general, acupuncture is a well-tolerated procedure, especially when done by a well-trained acupuncturist. The NIH panel that evaluated acupuncture stated: "the occurrence of adverse events ... has been documented to be extremely low"(1). The panel also concluded that acupuncture was "remarkably safe with fewer side effects than many well-established therapies." Mild side effects include bruising at acupuncture sites, needle pain, fatigue, and bleeding.

In one report, over a 20-year period, only 216 serious acupuncture-related complications were reported worldwide. Two other studies, each of which assessed about 30,000 acupuncture treatments, found no serious complications and approximately 40 minor side effects, such as nausea and fainting. Serious complications often are caused by poorly trained or negligent acupuncturists.

For people with MS, it is important to realize that acupuncture may produce drowsiness in up to one-third of people. This effect could conceivably be worse in people who have MS-associated fatigue or in those who take potentially sedating medication such as lioresal (Baclofen), tizanidine (Zanaflex), or diazepam (Valium).

Other rare risks are associated with acupuncture. Sterile disposable needles should be used to avoid hepatitis and AIDS. People with damaged or prosthetic heart valves should probably not be treated with acupuncture because of the risk of infection. People who take blood-thinning medication (warfarin or Coumadin) or who have bleeding disorders may occasionally experience bruising or, more rarely, bleeding complications.

Electroacupuncture may produce heart-rhythm abnormalities in people with a pacemaker, and the fumes from moxibustion may worsen breathing in people with asthma. Acupuncture to the chest should be done with caution or avoided to prevent lung or heart injury. These and other precautions of acupuncture are shown in Table 4.1.

Practical Information

Acupuncture usually is done once or twice weekly. Sessions typically last about 50 minutes and cost $60 to $200. The length of time required for a course of treatment varies. If a beneficial response occurs, it should usually be noted after six to ten sessions. The length of a complete course of treatment depends on the specific symptoms and the underlying disease process. A longer treatment course may be necessary for MS and other chronic diseases.

Approximately 10,000 licensed acupuncturists practice in the United States, 3,000 of whom have M.D. or D.O. training. Organizations that can be helpful in obtaining information about acupuncture and locating an acupuncturist include:

■ Acupuncture and Oriental Medicine Alliance (AOMA) , 6405 43rd Avenue Court. NW, Suite B, Gig Harbor WA 98335 (253-851-6896) (www.aomalliance.org)

TABLE 4.1. *Precautions with Acupuncture Use*

Avoid with:	Blood-thinning medication (warfarin or Coumadin) or bleeding disorder
	Damaged or prosthetic heart valves
	Pacemaker (electroacupuncture)
Use caution with:	Immune-suppressing drugs or conditions
	Pregnancy
	Metal allergy
	Acupuncture sites in thorax (risk of lung or heart injury)

- American Association of Acupuncture and Oriental Medicine, P.O. Box 162340, Sacramento CA 95816 (866-455-7999) (www.aaom.org)
- National Certification Commission for Acupuncture and Oriental Medicine 11 Canal Center Plaza, Suite 300, Alexandria VA 22314 (703-548-9004) (www.nccaom.org)
- A listing of physicians or osteopaths who have acupuncture training is available from the American Academy of Medical Acupuncture (800-521-2262) (www.medicalacupuncture.org)

Conclusion

Acupuncture usually is well tolerated, but rare adverse effects do occur. Variable results have been obtained in studies of MS and acupuncture. In small and preliminary studies, MS-associated symptoms that have responded to acupuncture include anxiety, depression, dizziness, pain (including headache, facial pain, low back pain, and neck pain), bladder difficulties, sleeping difficulties, and weakness.

Asian Proprietary Medicine (or Asian Patent Medicine)

Asian proprietary medicine, also known as Asian patent medicine, is a form of Asian herbal medicine. Preparations of this type of medicine usually contain mixtures of herbs as well as animal parts and minerals.

Several studies of the chemical composition of these preparations have found that they frequently contain potentially toxic ingredients. Recent data indicate that approximately one-third of these products contain drugs or dangerous metals. Drugs that have been found include diazepam (Valium), steroids, and prescription asthma medications. Toxic metals sometimes found in these products are arsenic, mercury, lead, and cadmium.

Because of the possible presence of these toxic ingredients, Asian proprietary medicine should be avoided or used with extreme caution.

Asian Herbal Medicine

Asian herbal medicine involves therapy using herbal preparations that are often complex mixtures of many different herbs. Asian herbal medicine frequently is used in combination with acupuncture, but it also may be used on its own. Asian herbal medicine may be administered in several different ways, including as tablets, pills, powders, capsules, or tinctures. Raw herbs or extracts of herbs also may be used.

When considering the use of Asian herbal medicine, it is essential to know which specific herbs are being used and to recognize that the full range of effectiveness and toxicity has not been fully established for any of these herbal preparations. These issues and other important factors related to herbal medicine in general are discussed in more detail in the section on herbs. In addition, the section on herbs has information on some Asian herbs, including Asian ginseng, astragalus, dong-quai, ephedra (*ma huang*), *Ginkgo biloba*, and licorice (see "Herbs").

Studies in MS and Other Conditions

Limited information is available on Asian herbal medicine in the treatment of MS. One study evaluated the effects of Ping Fu Tang, a mixture of 17 different herbs (8). In this study, 45 people with MS were monitored for nearly 3 years. Two groups were followed: a treatment group that received the herbal therapy, and a control group that was treated with conventional Western medicine or a combination of Western and Chinese medicine. The group that received the herbal therapy had a significant decrease in attack rate compared to the control group. Unfortunately, the results of this study are difficult to interpret because of limited reporting about the characteristics of the people in the study, the way in which the study was conducted, and the type of monitoring that was performed.

Several other studies of the use of Asian herbal medicine in MS have been reported. These studies are difficult to interpret because most of them have been published in Chinese and only summaries are readily available in English (9). In 1990, one Chinese study reported beneficial effects with herbal treatment in 35 people with MS. In 1995, another study reported by the same research group found that Ping Fu Tang, a mixture of 17 different herbs, decreased the rate of MS attacks. Several other MS studies of Chinese herbal medicine (as well as Japanese herbal medicine) have been conducted. Paradoxically, in one of these studies, an herb that appears to stimulate the immune system, *Ganoderma lucidum*, was reported to slow the disease course in five people with MS. Overall, because these studies are not available in English, it is impossible to rigorously evaluate them or to make any clear conclusions about the research results.

Several specific Chinese herbs have anti-inflammatory effects or suppress the activity of the immune system and therefore could be therapeutic for MS. These herbs include *Ginkgo biloba* (see "Herbs" chapter), Re Du Qing, Berberis, *Stephania tetrandra*, and *Tripterygium wilfordii*.

A compound from *Stephania tetrandra*, tetrandrine, has produced promising results in scientific studies. This chemical suppresses the immune system through mechanisms that are different from several conventional medications. In addition, tetrandrine appears to produce additional immune-suppressing effects when it is given in combination with conventional medications. One study showed that tetrandrine decreased the severity of experimental allergic encephalomyelitis (EAE), the animal model of MS. Further studies are needed to study the effects of this compound.

One of the more extensively studied immune-suppressing Chinese herbs is *Tripterygium wilfordii*, also known as Thunder God Vine, threewingnut, or lei-gong-teng. Scientific studies indicate that this herb decreases the activity of T cells and other specific components of the immune system. In addition, it lessens the severity of EAE. One study conducted in China following ten people with MS found that *T. wilfordii* produced "significant" improvement in eight people and mild improvement in two people.

T. wilfordii has been studied primarily in autoimmune disorders other than MS. Beneficial effects have been noted in animals with an experimental form of lupus. Some clinical improvement has been noted in people with rheumatoid arthritis and lupus.

At this time, studies are too limited for this therapy to be recommended specifically for MS or other autoimmune conditions. In addition, use of this herb has been associated with serious side effects (see below).

Side Effects

If considering Asian herbal medicine, people with MS should be aware of individual herbs or herbal mixtures that may stimulate the immune system (Table 4.2). The immune-stimulating effects of these herbs have been shown in scientific tests or in laboratory animals. Their effects on humans in general or on people with MS have not been specifically investigated. Thus, the immune-stimulating activity of the herbs represents a theoretical risk for people with MS.

Fu-zheng therapy, a type of Chinese herbal medicine, is believed to improve the ability of the body to defend itself. Two herbs used in Fu-zheng therapy, astragalus and *Ligustrum lucidum*, have been shown to activate immune cells. Licorice and Asian ginseng, which are present in many different types of Chinese herbal medicine, have diverse effects on the immune system, including stimulating effects. Green tea contains potent antioxidant compounds, which also may produce immune-stimulating activity; this is discussed elsewhere in this book (see "Coffee and Other Caffeine-Containing Herbs").

Some types of Japanese herbal medicine have immune-stimulating properties (see Table 4.2). Some of these mixtures also are used in Chinese

TABLE 4.2.   *Asian Herbal Medicine That May Stimulate the Immune System*

Chinese:	Asian ginseng (*Panax ginseng*)	Japanese:	Kakkan-to
	Acanthopanax obovatus		Kanzo-bushi-to
	Angelica sinensis (dong quai)		Shosaiko-to
	Artemisis myriantha		
	Artemisis annua		
	Astragalus (*Astragalus membranaceus*)		
	Coix		
	Epimedium sagittatum		
	Ge-gen-tang		
	Green tea		
	Licorice		
	Ligustrum lucidum		
	Maitake mushroom		
	Reishi mushroom (*Ganoderma lucidum*)		
	Salvia miltiorrhiza		
	Shiitake mushroom (*Lentinus edodes*)		
	Sophora flavescens		
	Xiao-chai-hu-tang		

medicine; for example, the Japanese herbs kakkan-to and shosaiko-to are the same as the Chinese herbs ge-gen-tang and xiao-chai-hu-tang, respectively.

Toxic effects have been associated with the use of some types of Asian herbal medicine (Table 4.3); these effects are not specific to MS. These herbs should be used with caution. Serious toxic effects on multiple body organs have been associated with some of these herbs. *T. wilfordii* has caused stomach upset, infertility, and, on one occasion, death. Less significant toxicity has been observed with the regular use of licorice, which may produce high blood pressure and low blood levels of potassium. The use of *ma huang* (ephedra) has been associated with increased blood pressure, other dangerous cardiac and neurologic side effects, and, rarely, death. Due to safety concerns, the FDA banned the sale of ephedra products in the United States on December 30, 2003.

TABLE 4.3.   *Potentially Toxic Asian Herbs*

Aristolochia fangchi	Guiji
Baijiaolia	Jin bu yuan
Bushi	Licorice
Caowu	*Ma huang* (ephedra)
Chuanwa	Naoyanghua
Datura preparations	*Tripterygium wilfordii*
Fuzi	Yangjinhua
Guangfangji	

Practical Information

Chinese herbal medicine should be obtained from a trained herbalist. Monthly costs are approximately $20 to $60.

Conclusion

On the basis of current evidence, acupuncture and Asian herbal medicine, both of which are components of traditional Chinese medicine (TCM), should be approached differently by people with MS. Acupuncture is of low risk, is possibly beneficial, and may be a reasonable treatment option for some people with MS. In contrast, Asian herbal medicine should be considered with caution by people with MS, especially for use on a long-term basis. Reports of treatment benefits using this therapy cannot be fully evaluated because of the lack of published information in English. Some herbs may be toxic or may stimulate the immune system, and the safety of long-term treatment has not generally been established.

Additional Resources

Books

Filshie J, White A. *Medical Acupuncture A Western Scientific Approach*. Edinburgh: Churchill Livingstone, 1998.

Freeman L. *Mosby's Complementary and Alternative Medicine: A Research-Based Approach*. St. Louis: Mosby, 2001, pp. 333–369.

Hsu DT, Cheng RL. Acupuncture. In: Weintraub MI, Micozzi MS, eds. *Alternative and Complementary Treatments in Neurologic Illness*. New York: Churchill Livingstone, 2001, pp. 11–26.

Lin Y-C. Acupuncture and traditional Chinese medicine. In: Oken BS, ed. *Complementary Therapies in Neurology*. London: Parthenon Publishing, 2004, pp. 113–125.

Navarra T. *The Encyclopedia of Complementary and Alternative Medicine*. New York: Checkmark Books. 2005, pp. 2–5.

Nielsen A, Hammerschlag R. Acupuncture and East Asian medicine. In: Kligler B, Lee R, eds. *Integrative Medicine: Principles for Practice*. New York: McGraw Hill, 2004, pp. 177–217.

Journal Articles

Borchers AT, Hackman RM, Keen CL, et al. Complementary medicine: A review of immunomodulatory effects of Chinese herbal medicines. *Am J Clin Nutrition* 1997;66:1303–1312.

Chan TYK, Critchley JAJH. Usage and adverse effects of Chinese herbal medicines. *Human Exp Toxicol* 1996;15:5–12.

Ho LJ, Lai JH. Chinese herbs as immunomodulators and potential disease-modify-ing antirheumatic drugs in autoimmune disorders. *Curr Drug Metab* 2004;5:181–192.

Lai JH. Immunomodulatory effects and mechanisms of plant alkaloid tetrandrine in autoimmune diseases. *Acta Pharmacol Sin* 2002;23:2093–1101.

Miller RE. An investigation into the management of the spasticity experienced by some patients with multiple sclerosis using acupuncture based on tradition-al Chinese medicine. *Compl Ther Med* 1996;4:58–62.

NIH Consensus Development Panel on Acupuncture. *JAMA* 1998;280:1518–1524.

Rabinstein AA, Shulman LM. Acupuncture in clinical neurology. *Neurologist* 2003;9:137–148.

Xi L, Zhiwen L, Huayan W, et al. Preventing relapse in multiple sclerosis with Chinese medicine. *J Chin Med* 2001;66:39–40.

Zhang L-H, Huang Y, Wang L-W, et al. Several compounds from Chinese tradi-tional and herbal medicine as immunomodulators. *Phytother Res* 1995;9:315–322.

5

Allergies

$\mathcal{A}$ long history of speculation exists concerning the association of multiple sclerosis (MS) with allergies. This idea was especially popular in the 1940s and 1950s. Many different allergic substances have been proposed over the years.

Various food allergies have been implicated in MS. Some studies have found that MS is more common in areas with high intakes of dairy products or gluten-containing grains, such as wheat, rye, oats, and barley. As a result, the consumption of dairy products or gluten has been implicated in MS. Other proposed allergic foods have included yeast, mushrooms and other fungi, fermented products (such as vinegar), sugar, potatoes, red meat, fruits, vegetables, caffeine, and tea and other tannin-containing foods.

Treatment Method

Several approaches may be taken to the treatment of allergies. If the allergic substance is a food, specific foods can be avoided. Another approach involves injecting the allergic substance under the skin; this leads to *desensitization*, which decreases the response to the allergic agent.

Studies in Multiple Sclerosis

A limited number of studies have evaluated the possible role of allergies in MS. No well-designed studies exist to support any specific food or environmental factor as an allergic cause of MS. In addition, no studies have demonstrated that eliminating exposure to a certain presumed allergic agent is beneficial.

One suspected allergic substance that has been investigated is *gluten*, a protein present in wheat and wheat products. However, studies of the intestinal lining and blood have not demonstrated a sensitivity to gluten in people with MS. Also, no benefit was found in a study of people with MS who did not consume gluten. In one study using the animal model of MS, a gluten-free diet actually *increased* the severity of the disease.

It is interesting to note that people with MS actually appear to have fewer allergic problems than do those who do not have the disease. Recent information indicates that people with MS have nearly 70 percent fewer allergic symptoms and more than 80 percent fewer positive allergy tests than the general population. This appears to be a result of the underlying immune disorder that occurs in MS.

In other studies, it appears that components of the immune system that are involved in allergies may play a role in MS. Specifically, *mast cells*, allergy-associated immune cells, are present in MS lesions in the central nervous system. In experimental allergic encephalomyelitis (EAE), the animal model of MS, brain lesions contain allergy-related immune cells and immune molecules. Also, in EAE, some studies show that disease severity is decreased when animals are treated with antihistamines and other compounds that inhibit the allergic response. In one study, antihistamine use was associated with a decreased risk of developing MS.

The role of allergic responses in MS is an evolving field. Although no evidence suggests that a specific allergy causes MS or that allergic responses are the primary immune abnormality in MS, it is possible that allergy-related components of the immune system may affect MS disease severity. These allergic components of the immune system are being studied as possible targets for future MS drug therapies.

Conclusion

At this time, no strong evidence suggests that MS is associated with an allergic response to a specific food or environmental factor. Based on a limited number of studies conducted in this area, there is no reason to believe that allergy-free diets or desensitization procedures are beneficial for patients with MS. Decreasing the activity of specific allergy-related immune processes may be a way to decrease MS disease severity—this area is currently being investigated as a novel treatment approach in MS.

Additional Readings

Journal Articles

Alonso A, Jick SS, Hernan MA. Allergy, histamine 1 receptor blockers, and the risk of multiple sclerosis. *Neurol* 2006;66:572–575.

DiMarco R, Mangano K, Quattrocchi C, et al. Exacerbation of protracted-relapsing experimental allergic encephalomyelitis in DA rats by gluten-free diets. *APMIS* 2004;112:651–655.

Hunter AL, Rees BW, Jones LT. Gluten antibodies in patients with multiple sclerosis. *Human Nutr-Appl Nutr* 1984;38:142–143.

Jones PE, Pallis C, Peters TJ. Morphological and biochemical findings in jejunal biopsies from patients with multiple sclerosis. *J Neurol Psych* 1979; 42:402–406.

Oro AS, Guarino TJ, Driver R, et al. Regulation of disease susceptibility: decreased prevalence of IgE-mediated allergic disease in patients with multiple sclerosis. *J Allergy Clin Immunol* 1996;97:1402–1408.

Pedotti R, DeVoss JJ, Youssef S, et al. Multiple elements of the allergic arm of the immune response modulate autoimmune demyelination. *Proc Natl Acad Sci USA* 2003;100:1867–1872.

Robbie-Ryan M, Brown M. The role of mast cells in allergy and autoimmunity. *Curr Opin Immunol* 2002;14:728–733.

Tang L, Benjaponpitak S, DeKruyff RH, et al. Reduced prevalence of allergic disease in patients with multiple sclerosis is associated with enhanced IL-12 production. *J Allergy Clin Immunol* 1998;102:428–435.

6

Aromatherapy

Aromatherapy is a type of healing that uses aromatic substances derived from plants. It was used in some form in ancient Egypt and ancient China. The type of aromatherapy currently used in the United States was originally developed in the early twentieth century by René-Maurice Gattefosse, a French chemist.

Treatment Method

Aromatherapy is based primarily on the use of essential oils. These oils, which are of high quality and purity, are obtained from plants using a specialized distillation process or by cold pressing. More than 40 different essential oils are used. They may be used individually or as mixtures, and they are administered by direct application to the skin, mixing with bath water, or inhalation. Oils sometimes are applied to the skin by massage. In France, oils are sometimes taken internally by mouth or by the vagina or rectum. However, in general, oils should not be taken internally.

As with the other senses, the sense of smell serves an important role. Specific odors may trigger feelings and memories. Some studies have shown that certain odors may produce headaches or elicit relaxation. The nerve signals from the nose are transmitted to a part of the brain known as the *limbic system*, which is involved in emotion and motivation.

Although smell often is thought of as a "minor" sense in humans, it is actually the major sense for many animals. For these animals, chemicals known as *pheromones* are detected by the olfactory system and are important in mating and communication.

Although the sense of smell is important, and olfactory signals are sent to a brain region involved in basic psychological processes, the mechanism by which administering certain odors may be therapeutic is not clear.

Studies in MS and Other Conditions

Aromatherapy has not been systematically studied in people with multiple sclerosis (MS). A small preliminary study of two people with MS reported that a treatment program of aromatherapy and massage led to improvement in mobility, dressing ability, and personal hygiene (1). Studies of olfaction in MS indicate that 10 to 20 percent of people with the disease have an impaired sense of smell.

Only a limited number of studies detail the effects of aromatherapy on any medical condition, and those that do exist are generally of low quality. Many of the therapeutic claims about aromatherapy are based on tradition, not on actual clinical research.

Symptoms of MS that have been investigated in some aromatherapy research are anxiety, depression, pain, and insomnia. For anxiety, studies of variable quality indicate that beneficial effects may be obtained with the use of lavender oil, Roman chamomile oil, and neroli (orange) oil. However, no large, well-designed clinical studies have examined this antianxiety effect. Preliminary information suggests that a lower dose of antidepressant medication may be needed by depressed men when the medication is used in combination with aromatherapy using a citrus fragrance. Lavender in bath water does not appear to relieve childbirth-associated pain. Positive and negative results have been obtained in other studies of aromatherapy and pain. Several fragrances, especially lavender, have been evaluated in sleep studies in animals and humans. Some positive results have been reported, but these studies are of variable quality.

Aromatherapy has been studied in a few other unrelated conditions. Small studies on older people with dementia have produced mixed results. Inhalation of black pepper extract may decrease the craving for cigarettes. People with a form of baldness called alopecia areata may benefit from scalp massage using a mixture of thyme, rosemary, lavender, and cedarwood oils.

When aromatherapy is combined with massage, as is often the case, it may be difficult to distinguish the benefits of the oil from those of the massage. In limited studies, massage alone has been associated with several beneficial effects (see the "Massage" chapter).

One author of an extensive review of aromatherapy and neurologic diseases concluded: "Having spent the last decade and a half investigating the scientific basis of aromatherapy and having published more than 100 peer-reviewed articles in this area, the author does not believe that scientific literature supports or that the risk/benefit ratio justifies use of aromatherapy in neurologic conditions at present. This is a fluid position, and as more studies are performed delineating the efficacy of aromatherapy, the author expects to endorse and use aromatherapy as part of the therapeutic armamentarium" (2).

Side Effects

Aromatherapy usually is well tolerated, but it is not risk-free. When applied to the skin, some oils may produce a skin rash (this type of allergic reaction may be detected by applying a small amount of oil to the skin and monitoring for a response for 24 hours). Cinnamon or clove oil should not be applied directly to the skin. Basil, fennel, lemon grass, rosemary, and verbena oils may cause skin irritation—the use of these oils should be discontinued if skin irritation occurs. Approximately 5 percent of people appear to be allergic to fragrances. Because of possible toxic effects, oil should not be taken internally by mouth or any other method (this is especially true for eucalyptus, hyssop, mugwort, thuja, pennyroyal, sage, and wormwood). Pregnant women probably should avoid aromatherapy because the use of some oils may lead to miscarriage. Odors may provoke headaches in people with migraines and cause breathing difficulties in those with asthma. Some oils (rosemary, fennel, hyssop, sage, wormwood) may cause seizures in people with epilepsy. Naphthalene-related compounds, such as menthol and camphor, should be avoided in those with a condition known as G6PD deficiency.

If aromatherapy is combined with massage, the possible side effects of massage should be kept in mind (see "Massage" chapter).

Practical Information

Aromatherapy may be obtained from a practitioner or may be self-administered. It is sometimes combined with herbal medicine or traditional Chinese medicine. Aromatherapy may be provided on an individual basis or as informational classes. Individual sessions typically cost $60 to $80 and last about 60 minutes. Classes cost about $30 for 60 to 120 minutes.

More information on aromatherapy and aromatherapists may be obtained from:

■ American Alliance of Aromatherapy, P.O. Box 309, Depoe Bay OR 93741 (800-809-9850)
■ Aromatherapy Registration Council (ARC) (www.aromatherapy-council.org)

■   National Association for Holistic Aromatherapy (NAHA)
    (www.naha.org), 3327 W. Indian Trail Road PMB 144, Spokane WA
    99208 (509-325-3419)

Conclusion

Aromatherapy is of low risk and reasonable cost. The benefits of this
therapy in people with MS have not been systematically studied. A small,
preliminary study in MS found improvement in multiple symptoms using
aromatherapy and massage. Some small clinical studies have found beneficial effects for anxiety, depression, pain, and insomnia, but these studies
are of variable quality and some of the results have not been consistent.
One large study found that aromatherapy was not effective for pain.
Further research is needed on the effects of aromatherapy on MS and other
neurologic conditions.

Additional Readings

Books

Ernst E, ed. *The Desktop Guide to Complementary and Alternative Medicine: An
    Evidence-Based Approach.* Edinburgh: Mosby, 2001, pp.33–35.
Fugh-Berman A. *Alternative Medicine: What Works.* Baltimore: Williams & Wilkins,
    1997, pp. 182–187.
Hirsh AR. Aromatherapy: art, science, or myth? In: Weintraub MI, Micozzi M, eds.
    Alternative and Complementary Treatment in Neurologic Illness. Philadelphia:
    Churchill Livingstone, 2001, pp. 128–150.
Kowalak JP, Mills EJ, eds. *Professional Guide to Complementary and Alternative
    Therapies.* Springhouse, PA: Springhouse Publishing, 2001, pp. 52–53.
Navarra T. *The Encyclopedia of Complementary and Alternative Medicine.* New York:
    Checkmark Books. 2005, pp.8–10.
Vickers A. *Massage and Aromatherapy: A Guide for Health Professionals.* London:
    Chapman & Hall, 1996.

Journal Articles

Howarth AL. Will aromatherapy be a useful treatment strategy for people with
    multiple sclerosis who experience pain? *Compl Ther Nurs Midwifery* 2002;
    8:138–141.
Walsh E, Wilson C. Complementary therapies in long-stay neurology in-patient
    settings. *Nursing Standard* 1999;13:32–35.

7

Aspartame

Some claims exist that aspartame, an artificial sweetener used in soft drinks, causes multiple sclerosis (MS) or worsens MS-associated symptoms.

Treatment Method

It sometimes is recommended that people with MS avoid all drinks and foods that contain aspartame. It also sometimes is suggested that stevia, an herbal, non-sugar sweetener (also known as sweetleaf) be used instead of sugar or aspartame. Stevia contains stevioside, a chemical that is about 300 times sweeter than sugar (sucrose).

Studies in MS and Other Conditions

No well-conducted studies have shown that aspartame causes MS or worsens symptoms in most people with the disease. Through www.ms-cam.org, the CAM website of the Rocky Mountain Multiple Sclerosis Center, we conducted a survey of aspartame use among a large group of people with MS. We had 3,075 people with MS respond to this survey. A minority (15 percent) of those who responded experienced problems that they attributed to aspartame use. Headache was the most common complaint, which was noted by about one third (36 percent) of those who noticed symptoms related to aspartame. Among MS symptoms, those that were reported to be worsened most commonly by aspartame were fatigue, thinking problems, weakness, and numbness. Nearly two-thirds of people reported that their aspartame-related symptoms began within minutes or hours of using the sweetener. Overall, these findings indicate that the majority of people with MS do not have problems with aspartame and that the most common symptom provoked by aspartame, headache, is not an MS-specific symptom. The full results of this survey may be viewed on the website, www.ms-cam.org.

Limited studies indicate that aspartame may provoke migraine headaches and worsen depression. Interestingly, one migraine medication that dissolves in the mouth, known as rizatriptan or Maxalt-MLT, actually contains aspartame and may worsen headache in those with aspartame-provoked migraines. In terms of other neurologic disorders, clinical studies do not indicate that aspartame worsens Parkinson's disease or epilepsy.

Aspartame is of potential concern because the body may convert aspartame to methanol and then convert the methanol to formic acid, which may produce serious toxicity. However, consuming moderate or even large quantities of diet soft drinks does not significantly increase blood levels of methanol or formic acid.

Side Effects

Limited safety information is available for stevia, the herbal sweetener. Stevia may cause nausea and abdominal fullness. It also may decrease blood sugar levels and may decrease blood pressure. Other possible side effects include headache, dizziness, myalgia, and numbness. Stevia may cause allergic reactions in people who are allergic to plants in the Asteraceae/Compositae family, which includes daisies, marigold, ragweed, and chrysanthemums. The safety of long-term stevia use is not known. In the United States, although the Food and Drug Administration (FDA) allows stevia to be imported as a dietary supplement, it is classified as an "unsafe food additive" due to the limited safety information.

Conclusion

Given the limited results that are available at this time, no compelling reason exists for most people with MS to avoid aspartame. There is no strong evidence that a reasonable intake of aspartame worsens MS or provokes MS-associated symptoms. A subgroup of people with MS may experience aspartame-related symptoms. To determine if one is in this subgroup, it would be reasonable to discontinue aspartame use for a few days and note if any benefit occurs.

Additional Resources

Books

Jellin JM, Batz F, Hitchens K. *Natural Medicines Comprehensive Database.* Stockton, CA: Therapeutic Research Faculty, 2005, pp. 1176–1178.

Journal Articles

Leon AS, Hunninghake DB, Bell C, et al. Safety of long-term doses of aspartame. *Arch Int Med* 1989;149:2318–2324.

Lipton RB, Newman LC, Cohen JS, et al. Aspartame as a dietary trigger of headache. *Headache* 1989;29:90–92.

Newman LC, Lipton RB. Maxalt MLT-down: an unusual presentation of migraine in patients with aspartame-triggered headaches. *Headache* 2001;41:899–901.

Van dewn Eeden SK, Koepsell TD, Longstreth WT Jr., et al. Aspartame ingestion and headaches: a randomized crossover trial. *Neurology* 1994;44:1787–1793.

Walton RG, Hudak R, Green-Waite RJ. Adverse reactions to aspartame: double-blind challenge in patients from a vulnerable population. *Biol Psych* 1993;34:13–17.

8

Ayurveda

*A*yurveda was developed in India thousands of years ago and is the oldest known medical system still in use. Ayurveda means "knowledge (or science) of life" in Sanskrit, and its practice includes medicine and science as well as philosophy and religion. The form of Ayurvedic medicine now practiced is a modified version of the ancient form of this healing method. Ayurveda is still widely practiced in India. It has been popularized and promoted in the United States by Maharishi Mahesh Yogi and Dr. Deepak Chopra.

In Ayurveda, a harmonious relationship between mind, body, and spiritual awareness is believed to be important. The function of these entities is regulated by three physiologic principles known as doshas. Disease is claimed to be the result of an imbalance of the *doshas*, and treatment aims to restore dosha balance. As in traditional Chinese medicine, Ayurveda holds that an important life force, called *prana*, exists.

Treatment Method

Ayurveda consists of several components. As in traditional Chinese medicine, pulse and tongue evaluation are important for diagnosis. Diet, exercise, lifestyle changes, and specific supplements are used therapeutically. Yoga, breathing exercises, massage, and meditation, discussed elsewhere in this book, are also components of Ayurveda. One type of Ayurvedic meditation, transcendental meditation (TM), was popularized by Maharishi Mahesh Yogi. Another important aspect of Ayurveda, *panchakarma*, is used for disease prevention. Panchakarma means "five processes" and includes massages, sweat baths, vomiting, enemas, and bloodletting (through the use of leeches).

One specific Ayurvedic supplement, known as *ashwagandha*, is sometimes specifically recommended for treating multiple sclerosis (MS). This supplement is derived from the roots of the *Withania somnifera* plant.

Two primary types of Ayurveda are practiced outside India. Maharishi Ayur-Veda was started by Maharishi Mahesh Yogi and relies heavily on meditation. The other Ayurvedic school, advocated by Dr. Deepak Chopra, uses meditation in conjunction with other Ayurvedic methods.

Studies in MS and Other Conditions

No large published clinical studies have specifically investigated the effect of Ayurveda on MS or its symptoms. Some components of Ayurveda have been investigated individually. These include massage, meditation, and yoga, all of which are discussed elsewhere in this book. These therapies may be helpful for some symptoms that occur with MS, including fatigue, spasticity, pain, depression, and anxiety.

Ashwagandha, the Ayurvedic supplement sometimes recommended for MS, has been studied mainly in scientific and animal studies. In these studies, ashwagandha has been shown to stimulate the immune system. It also may produce sedating effects. Ashwagandha has not been studied in clinical trials in MS—as a result, it is not known if it has any therapeutic effects in MS.

Some research has evaluated Ayurvedic supplements for other conditions. One small study found that the herb *Phyllanthus* was an effective therapy for liver inflammation; subsequent studies did not find beneficial effects. For asthma, mixed results have been obtained using an Ayurvedic preparation, *Tylophora indica asthmatica*. In experimental animal models of breast and lung cancer, beneficial effects have been shown for Maharishi-4, also known as Maharishi Amrit Kalash-4 or MAK-4. Curcumin, MA-631, and Maharishi-5, produce biochemical effects that might be beneficial for heart disease.

Research on Ayurveda currently is being conducted collaboratively. The National Institute of Ayurvedic Medicine (NIAM) is doing research in conjunction with the National Cancer Institute (Bethesda, MD), the Central Council for Research in Ayurveda and Siddha Medicine (New Delhi, India), the Mount Sinai School of Medicine (New York, NY), and the Richard and Hinda Rosenthal Center for Alternative and Complementary Medicine at Columbia University (New York, NY). NIAM currently is conducting studies on the effects of panchakarma therapies on the immune system.

Side Effects

Ayurveda should not be used in place of conventional medicine for treating MS. Some Ayurvedic preparations contain dangerous heavy metals, such as lead, arsenic, and mercury. These preparations have been associated with serious metal poisoning and should be avoided, even if they are claimed to be "deactivated" by heat. One study of 70 different Ayurvedic herbal preparations found that 20 percent contained potentially harmful levels of certain metals.

Ashwagandha sometimes is recommended for MS. However, due to its immune-stimulating effects, this Ayurvedic supplement poses theoretical risks for people with MS. These effects also could interfere with the effectiveness of the FDA-approved injectable medications for MS (glatiramer acetate [Copaxone], interferons [Avonex, Betaseron, and Rebif]), natalizumab (Tysabri), and chemotherapy drugs that are sometimes used to treat MS, such as methotrexate, azathioprine (Imuran), mitoxantrone (Novantrone), and mycophenolate (CellCept). The sedating effects of ashwagandha could worsen MS fatigue or increase the sedating effects of some medications. Ashwagandha may interfere with thyroid and blood-thinning medications.

Scientific studies indicate that other Ayurvedic supplements also influence the immune system. Immune-stimulating activity has been noted in isolated scientific studies of Maharishi-4, Maharishi-5, *Boerhavia diffusa, Phyllanthus emblica*, and *Nimba arishta*. These preparations theoretically could be harmful to people with MS; clinical studies are needed to determine if they are in fact dangerous.

Ayurvedic remedies containing *Heliotropium* species have been associated with liver toxicity, which in some cases has led to death. Chemicals that may produce liver or kidney toxicity have been found in several Ayurvedic herbs, including *Cassia auriculata, Crotolaria juncea, Crotolaria verrucosa*, and *Holorrhena antidysenterica*. Kidney or liver toxicity in animals has been associated with *Aegle marmelos, Hemidesmus indicus, Terminalis chebula*, and *Withania somnifera*.

Practical Information

No program is in place for licensing Ayurvedic practitioners in the United States. Ayurveda is practiced by a variety of health care professionals, including physicians, chiropractors, and nutritionists. Initial visits with Ayurvedic practitioners last 1 to 3 hours; follow-up visits are 30 to 60 minutes. The initial evaluation costs between $90 and $225, and follow-up visits cost $60 to $90. Ayurveda usually is not covered by insurance. More information about Ayurveda and Ayurvedic medical practices may be obtained from local libraries and health food stores. Associations that provide information include:

- The American School of Ayurvedic Sciences, 2115 112th Avenue NE, Bellevue WA 98004 (425-453-8022)
- Ayurvedic Institute (www.ayurveda.com), 11311 Menaul Boulevard NE, Albuquerque NM 87112 (505-291-9698)

Conclusion

Ayurveda is a multicomponent healing system with generally low risk and moderate cost. Some components of Ayurveda, including massage, meditation, and yoga, are of low risk and may provide beneficial effects for fatigue, anxiety, depression, pain, and spasticity. However, another component of Ayurveda, the use of specific supplements, may produce serious side effects. This aspect of Ayurvedic treatment has not been fully studied in any medical condition, including MS. Ashwagandha, a specific Ayurvedic supplement sometimes recommended for MS, actually poses theoretical risks for people with MS because it could worsen the disease, decrease the therapeutic effects of some MS medications, and worsen MS fatigue or increase the sedating effects of some medications.

The overall assessment of Ayurveda is similar to that of traditional Chinese medicine. Both of these multicomponent healing methods may provide beneficial effects through *some* of their approaches, such as acupuncture and t'ai chi in traditional Chinese medicine and massage, meditation, and yoga in Ayurveda. These approaches may be worth considering for some people with MS. However, the biologically based components of both of these healing systems, which are herbal medicine in traditional Chinese medicine and supplements in Ayurveda, are generally of unknown safety and effectiveness, may pose theoretical risks in MS, and thus should be used with caution by people with MS.

Additional Readings

Books

Fetrow CW, Avila JR. *Complementary and Alternative Medicines*. Philadelphia: Lippincott, Williams, and Wilkins, 2004, pp. 58–60.

Jellin JM, Batz F, Hitchens K. *Natural Medicines Comprehensive Database*. Stockton, CA: Therapeutic Research Faculty, 2005, pp. 82–83.

Kaplan GP. Ayurvedic medicine. In: Oken BS, ed. *Complementary Therapies in Neurology*. London: Parthenon Publishing, 2004, pp. 145–158.

Manyam BV. Ayurvedic approach to neurologic illness. In: Weintraub MI, Micozzi MS, eds. *Alternative and Complementary Treatment in Neurologic Illness*. New York: Churchill Livingstone. 2001, pp. 68–74.

Navarra T. *The Encyclopedia of Complementary and Alternative Medicine.* New York: Checkmark Books. 2005, p. 13.

Pai S, Shanbhag V, Archarya S. Ayurvedic medicine. In: Kligler B, Lee R, eds. *Integrative Medicine: Principles for Practice.* New York: McGraw-Hill, 2004, pp. 219–240.

Journal Articles

Agarwal R, Diwanay S, Patki P, et al. Studies on immunomodulatory activity of Withania somnifera (Ashwagandha) extracts in experimental immune inflammation. *J Ethnopharmacol* 1999;67:27–35.

Iuvone T, Esposito G, Capasso F, et al. Induction of nitric oxide synthase expression by Withania somnifera in macrophages. *Life Sci* 2003;72:1617–1625.

Saper RB, Kales SN, Paquin J, et al. Heavy metal content of Ayurvedic herbal medicine products. *JAMA* 2004;292:2868–2873.

Ziauddin M, Phansalkar N, Patki P, et al. Studies on the immunomodulatory effects of Ashwagandha. *J Ethnopharmacol* 1996;50:69–76.

9

Bee Venom Therapy and Other Forms of Apitherapy

Bee venom therapy, used by some people with multiple sclerosis (MS), is one type of *apitherapy*. This term refers to the use of bees or bee products to treat medical conditions. It is estimated that 5,000 to 10,000 people with MS in the United States use bee venom therapy.

Apitherapy has been used for thousands of years. It was used in ancient Egypt. In ancient Greece, Hippocrates used bee venom to treat arthritis. Bee venom therapy has been used by famous leaders, including Charlemagne, Ivan the Terrible, and Charles the Great.

In more recent times, apitherapy, especially bee venom therapy, has been recommended by some people for MS and other autoimmune conditions, such as rheumatoid arthritis, lupus, and scleroderma. In the United States, Charles Mraz, also known as "The Bee Man," first advocated bee venom therapy during the 1930s. He initially treated his own arthritis effectively using bee venom therapy and subsequently recommended the treatment to people with arthritis and other inflammatory conditions, including MS. He claimed that the bee sting produces inflammation at the site of the sting and that the body then mounts an anti-inflammatory response. This anti-inflammatory response is believed to act not only against the sting but also against other inflammatory processes in the body.

Another popular recent advocate of bee venom therapy is Pat Wagner, known as "The Bee Lady." She has MS and claims to have used bee venom therapy effectively to treat herself.

Bee Venom Therapy

A variety of insects, collectively referred to as "bees," may inject venom through a burning sting. Honeybees generally are used in bee venom therapy.

Along with wasps, yellow jackets, and hornets, honeybees are species in a family of insects known as Hymenoptera.

The venom of bees is produced by specialized cells. It has two purposes: to defend against attackers and to weaken or paralyze prey. Bee venom contains a mixture of substances. The pain and swelling that result from a bee sting are produced by chemicals, including histamine, dopamine, norepinephrine, and serotonin. Bee venom also contains several toxins that are known as apamin, melittin, mast-cell degranulating peptide, and monamine. Finally, bee venom contains proteins that are involved in allergic responses. These proteins (including phospholipase-A2 and hyaluronidase) activate some immune cells and stimulate the production of one specific type of antibody, immunoglobulin E (IgE).

Bee venom contains many different substances. At this time, it is not known exactly how each of these substances interacts with the body and what effect they might have on a disease process such as MS.

Treatment Method

In bee venom therapy, a bee usually is grasped with tweezers and put on a particular part of the body. Tweezers then are used to remove the stinger 10 to 15 minutes after the sting. Ice sometimes is used on the skin before and after the sting to decrease the pain. Bee venom therapy typically is done in three sessions each week, and 20 to 40 stings are done in each session.

Studies in MS and Other Conditions

Experimental studies indicate that the components of bee venom have biologic effects that could affect an inflammatory disease such as MS. Various mixtures of multiple venom proteins produced anti-inflammatory effects in one study. Other studies have shown that two specific components of venom, melittin and adolapin, also have anti-inflammatory properties. In contrast, other studies have shown that bee venom components actually cause an inflammatory response. Also, apamin, a chemical constituent of the venom, has some effects that could be beneficial for MS. Apamin inhibits the action of a component of the nerve cell known as the *potassium channel*. This is the same part of the nerve cell affected by the experimental drug 4AP (4-aminopyridine), which may be beneficial for MS-associated fatigue. However, it is not clear that bee venom therapy produces high enough levels of apamin in the central nervous system to significantly inhibit potassium channels. Further studies are needed in this area.

To attempt to determine the effect of bee venom on MS, studies have been undertaken using experimental allergic encephalomyelitis (EAE), an animal form of MS. In these studies, mice with EAE were injected with honeybee venom three times weekly (1). Each injection was equivalent to 4 to 160 bee stings. Treatment with venom produced no benefit. In fact, in some animals, venom treatment may have produced a worsening of symptoms, relative to those that received a placebo.

Bee venom therapy has been evaluated in humans. Isolated accounts exist of individuals with MS who improved after this treatment. In the late 1990s, a study of the safety of bee venom therapy in humans began at Georgetown University. The results of this study have not been published. A more recent study, conducted in 2004 in The Netherlands, is the highest quality study to date (2). In this clinical trial, a *randomized crossover study*, 26 people with relapsing-remitting or secondary-progressive MS were randomly assigned to receive either no treatment or bee venom therapy for 24 weeks. After this initial phase, people "crossed over" to the other treatment method for another 24 weeks—that is, those who received no treatment were then treated with bee venom therapy and those who received bee venom therapy then received no treatment. Detailed clinical and MRI measures were used to monitor people during the study. No beneficial effects were found in terms of various MRI measures, numbers of attacks, neurologic disability, fatigue, and overall quality of life. Bee venom therapy was generally well tolerated.

Side Effects

In general, bee venom therapy is well tolerated. The most common side effect is swelling and redness at the sting site. About 20 percent of people experience itching, hives, fatigue, or anxiety. Women appear to have more frequent and severe side effects than do men. In the recent clinical trial of bee venom therapy in The Netherlands, no severe side effects were noted (2). Mild side effects included itching, flulike symptoms, and tenderness, swelling, and redness near sting sites.

Death is a very rare, but obviously important, adverse effect. Approximately 40 cases of bee sting deaths occur annually in the United States. Bee sting deaths frequently are attributed entirely to severe allergic reactions (anaphylaxis), but many of these deaths actually may be due to heart attacks that occur as a result of the stress of a mild allergic reaction in combination with heat, dehydration, or underlying heart disease. Importantly, severe allergic reactions may occur in individuals who have no past history of reactions to bee stings. Because of the possibility of a severe allergic reaction, a bee sting kit (Epi-Pen Autoinjector) should be available if bee venom therapy is used.

People with MS should be aware of another rare side effect of bee venom therapy: inflammation of the central nervous system similar to that which occurs in MS. One form of inflammation that has been associated with bee stings, known as *acute disseminated encephalomyelitis* (ADEM), involves multiple areas in the brain and spinal cord. Another specific type of inflammation associated with bee stings is *optic neuritis*. This condition involves inflammation of the nerve that connects the eye to the brain. Optic neuritis may produce mild or severe impairment of vision and is one of the more common conditions caused by MS. There have been reports of stings on or near the eye producing an MS-like form of optic neuritis in people who do not have MS. It is sometimes recommended that bee stings be given to the temple or eyebrows for visual problems. It would be safest for people with MS (and people without MS) to *avoid bee stings in this area* because of the possibility of bee sting–induced optic neuritis.

Finally, it is important to note that no formal studies have evaluated the long-term safety of bee venom therapy. As a result, it is not known if chronic bee venom therapy use is associated with significant toxic effects that have yet to be identified.

Other Bee Products

A variety of bee products other than bee venom also are used in apitherapy. These products often are recommended for MS and those symptoms that may occur with the disease, such as fatigue, weakness, visual difficulties, and memory problems. No evidence suggests that these products are effective for MS or MS-associated symptoms.

Bee Pollen

Bee pollen, which is composed of plant pollens, plant nectars, and bee saliva, is sometimes recommended to lessen fatigue, increase strength, and improve many other ailments. It contains a variety of nutrients, but it also may be contaminated with rodent debris, bacteria, insects, and the eggs and feces of insects. Rarely, bee pollen may cause severe allergic reactions, especially in those with pollen allergies. Asthma may worsen after bee pollen use. Isolated reports suggest that liver toxicity may be associated with bee pollen. Pollen could increase the risk of liver toxicity associated with some MS medications, such as interferons and methotrexate. Studies of bee pollen use in college and high school athletes have not demonstrated improvement in physical performance. There are no clear reasons for consuming bee pollen because it has no clear therapeutic properties and may have adverse effects.

Propolis

Propolis, a waxlike material also known as "bee glue," is collected by bees from buds on poplar and conifer trees and is used to repair cracks in hives. It may be weakly effective in killing a variety of bacteria and viruses. Limited studies have shown both stimulation and suppression of immune system activity. Propolis may facilitate the healing of mouth lesions and genital herpes lesions. One component of propolis, caffeic acid phenethyl ester (CAPE), has anti-inflammatory effects and, in one study, decreased the severity of disease in EAE, the animal model of MS. Whether propolis has an effect on MS is not known—no published clinical studies have been undertaken of propolis use in MS. No studies have systematically examined the safety of propolis use. Propolis may cause allergic reactions, especially in people with allergies to bees or bee products.

Raw Honey

It is sometimes claimed that honey contains valuable minerals and vitamins. Actually, honey contains approximately 80 percent sugar and 20 percent water. The mineral and vitamin content of honey is very low. Honey applied to the skin may improve healing from burns. No clinical studies have been undertaken of honey use in MS. Honey consumption is generally safe.

Royal Jelly

Royal jelly is recommended for many conditions, including some MS-associated symptoms such as weakness, depression, cognitive difficulties, and sexual problems. Royal jelly is a white substance produced by worker bees and is important in the development of queen bees. It has many chemical constituents, including neopterin, which is a compound secreted by immune system cells, and royalisin, a protein that has antibiotic activity. As with propolis, a small number of studies suggest that royal jelly may activate or suppress the immune system. No clinical studies exist of royal jelly use in MS. Royal jelly may provoke asthma; in one case, royal jelly was associated with a fatal asthma attack. Royal jelly use also has been associated with allergic reactions, including nasal congestion, itching, hives, and severe breathing difficulties (anaphylaxis). People with asthma or significant allergies should use royal jelly with caution.

Practical Information

Anyone considering bee venom therapy should first discuss it with a physician. For possible allergic reactions, it is important to have a bee sting kit available and to know how to use it. The names of local beekeepers can be obtained from the U.S. Department of Agriculture. Other bee products are available in pharmacies, health food stores, and apitherapy specialty stores.

Conclusion

No well-documented benefits have been noted for the use of bee venom therapy and other bee products for people with MS. One well-designed study of bee venom therapy in MS did not find any benefits in terms of various MRI and clinical measures. In addition, this type of treatment produces rare, but potentially serious, adverse effects, which include severe allergic reactions and death with bee venom therapy, and allergic reactions and worsening of asthma with the use of other bee products.

Additional Readings

Books

Cassileth BR. *The Alternative Medicine Handbook*. New York: W.W. Norton, 1998:155–158.

Fetrow CW, Avila JR. *Professional's Handbook of Complementary and Alternative Medicines*. Philadelphia: Lippincott, Williams, and Wilkins. 2004, pp. 79–81, 718–720.

Jellin JM, Batz F, Hitchens K. *Natural Medicines Comprehensive Database*. Stockton, CA: Therapeutic Research Faculty, 2005, pp. 103–104, 681–683, 1034–1035, 1088–1089.

Kowalak JP, Mills EJ, eds. *Professional Guide to Complementary and Alternative Therapies*. Springhouse, PA: Springhouse Publishing, 2001, pp. 47–48.

Journal Articles

Boz C, Velioglu S, Ozmenoglu M. Acute disseminated encephalomyelitis after bee sting. *Neurol Sci* 2003;23:313–315.

Ilhan A, Akyol O, Gurel A, et al. Protective effects of caffeic phenethyl ester against experimental allergic encephalomyelitis-induced oxidative stress in rats. *Free Radic Biol Med* 2004;37:386–394.

Lublin FD, Oshinsky RJ, Perreault, M, et al. Effect of honey bee venom on EAE. *Neurology* 1998;50:A424.

Nam KW, Je KH, Lee JH, et al. Inhibition of COX-2 activity and proinflammatory cytokines (TNF-alpha and IL-1beta) production by water-soluble sub-fractionated parts from bee (*Apis mellifera*) venom. *Arch Pharm Res* 2003; 26:383–388.

Song H-S, Wray SH. Bee sting optic neuritis. *J Clin Neuro-opth* 1991;11:45–49.

Wesselius T, Heersema DJ, Mostert JP, et al. A randomized crossover study of bee sting therapy for multiple sclerosis. *Neurology* 2005;65:1764–1768.

10

Biofeedback

Biofeedback uses the mind–body connection for therapeutic purposes. Biofeedback involves the use of machines to monitor bodily functions such as heart rate, pulse, or muscle tension. An individual undergoing biofeedback attempts to consciously alter one of these presumably "involuntary" bodily processes. The use of biofeedback has been investigated for many medical conditions.

Treatment Method

In biofeedback, monitoring equipment is used to translate the activity of specific bodily functions into images or sounds. The images may be seen on a computer screen or the sounds may be heard. The monitoring methods that are used depend on which physiologic activity is of interest: electromyography (EMG) biofeedback is used to monitor muscle tension; thermal biofeedback to monitor skin temperature; electrodermal response to monitor perspiration; respiration biofeedback to monitor the rate, rhythm, and volume of breathing; finger pulse biofeedback to monitor pulse rate; and brainwave biofeedback to monitor brain electrical activity.

During a biofeedback session, a biofeedback therapist assists an individual in altering the activity of a particular body process through mental or physical exercises. The individual learns methods to produce the desired change through feedback from the monitor, input from the therapist, and experimentation. These methods eventually can be used without the use of monitoring equipment.

Studies in MS and Other Conditions

Biofeedback may have applications for multiple sclerosis (MS)-related symptoms. For anxiety and insomnia, which may be significant problems in MS, biofeedback may be beneficial by promoting relaxation. It also may be helpful in treating some types of pain, including tension headaches, migraines, and low back pain. However, the use of biofeedback to treat MS-associated pain has not been formally studied.

Some research suggests that biofeedback may be helpful for people with urinary incontinence, a problem that may occur in MS. Medications and pelvic exercises are available for incontinence. These approaches may not be fully effective, however, and the medications may have undesirable side effects. Studies for biofeedback treatment of urinary incontinence have reported mixed results. Biofeedback may be especially effective for people who have difficulty knowing which muscles to contract during the performance of pelvic exercises. Studies must be done to more fully evaluate biofeedback therapy for urinary incontinence, specifically for MS-related urinary incontinence.

People with MS also may experience bowel incontinence. Biofeedback may be beneficial for this problem. In people with bowel incontinence related to conditions other than MS, biofeedback produces improvement in approximately 70 percent. In a small study of the effects of biofeedback on 15 people with MS-related constipation or stool incontinence, five showed improvement. Those who benefited from biofeedback had mild to moderate disability and had relatively stable disease during the time of treatment.

Finally, MS may produce *spasticity*, or stiffness in the arms and legs. Some studies in people with cerebral palsy indicate that spasticity may respond to biofeedback, but no large studies specifically addressing MS-associated spasticity have been done.

An interesting issue is whether biofeedback may be used to regulate the immune system and, conceivably, thereby alter immune diseases such as MS. Variable effects of biofeedback-induced relaxation on immune function have been obtained; no consistent results have been reported.

Biofeedback may be an effective treatment for many other conditions. Biofeedback may improve circulation, mildly decrease blood pressure, and be beneficial for alcoholism, drug abuse, and posttraumatic stress disorder.

Side Effects

Biofeedback usually is very well tolerated. In the case of electrodermal biofeedback, people with heart conditions and pacemakers should be cautious and should discuss the treatment with their physician. Biofeedback should be done with medical supervision in those with psychosis or severe personality disorders. Biofeedback may occasionally cause anxiety, dizziness, disorientation, and floating sensations.

Practical Information

Biofeedback should be obtained from a trained therapist. Self-operated biofeedback devices are available, but biofeedback monitoring is a complex process that is most likely to be helpful when it is performed by a qualified practitioner. Biofeedback sessions typically last 30 to 60 minutes. The number of sessions required ranges from a few to 30 or 40. Health insurance sometimes provides coverage for this therapy.

Many trained biofeedback therapists are psychologists. Certification is provided by the Biofeedback Certification Institute of America. Biofeedback practitioners can be found in the telephone directory under psychologists or by obtaining a directory of biofeedback therapists from the Biofeedback Certification Institute of America (www.bcia.org), 10200 W. 44th Avenue, Suite 310, Wheat Ridge, CO 80033 (303-420-2902). An organization that provides biofeedback information and is involved in biofeedback research is the Association for Applied Psychophysiology and Biofeedback (www.aapb.org), 10200 W. 44th Avenue, Suite 304, Wheat Ridge, CO 80033 (303-422-8894).

Conclusion

Biofeedback is a low-risk, moderate-cost therapy that may be beneficial for some MS-associated conditions. It may be especially helpful in those situations in which conventional medical approaches are not fully effective or produce side effects. MS symptoms that may be responsive to biofeedback include anxiety, insomnia, pain, urinary incontinence, fecal incontinence, and muscle stiffness. Further studies are needed to fully evaluate the effectiveness of biofeedback for MS symptoms.

Additional Readings

Books

Cassileth BR. *The Alternative Medicine Handbook*. New York: W.W. Norton, 1998, pp. 117–121.

Ernst E, ed. *The Desktop Guide to Complementary and Alternative Medicine: An Evidence-Based Approach*. Edinburgh: Mosby, 2001, pp. 40–42.

Fugh-Berman A. *Alternative Medicine: What Works*. Baltimore: Williams & Wilkins, 1997, pp. 41–46.

McGrady A. Biofeedback in the neurologic disorders. In: Weintraub MI, Micozzi MS, eds. *Alternative and Complementary Treatment in Neurologic Illness*. New York: Churchill Livingstone. 2001, pp. 156–165.

Journal Articles

Berghmans LCM, Hendriks HJM, Hay-Smith EJ, et al. Conservative treatment of stress urinary incontinence in women: a systematic review of randomized clinical trials. *Br J Urol* 1998;82:181–191.

Cattaneo D, Ferrarin M, Frasson W, et al. Head control: volitional aspects of rehabilitation training in patients with multiple sclerosis compared with healthy subjects. *Arch Phys Med Rehabil* 2005;86:1381–1388.

de Kruif YP, van Wegen Erwin EH. Pelvic floor muscle exercise therapy with myofeedback for women with stress urinary incontinence: a meta-analysis. *Physiotherapy* 1996;82:107–113.

Klarskov P, Heely E, Nyholdt I, et al. Biofeedback treatment of bladder dysfunction in multiple sclerosis. A randomized trial. *Scand J Urol Nephrol Suppl* 1994; 157:61–65.

Norton C, Hosker G, Brazzelli M. Biofeedback and/or sphincter exercises for the treatment of faecal incontinence in adults (Cochrane review). In: The Cochrane Library, Issue 2, 2000. Oxford: Update Software.

Wiesel PH, Norton C, Roy AJ, et al. Gut focused behavioural treatment (biofeedback) for constipation and faecal incontinence in multiple sclerosis. *J Neurol Neurosurg Psychiatry* 2000;69:240–243.

11

Candida Treatment

$\mathcal{M}$ultiple sclerosis (MS) has been associated with *Candida* infections, which are caused by a species of yeast. The most common type of *Candida* is *Candida albicans*. Mild infections with *Candida* may involve the mouth, which is referred to as *thrush*, or the vagina, which is referred to as *monilia*. More significant infections with *Candida* usually occur in people with conditions that suppress the immune system, such as AIDS and the use of chemotherapy medications. These infections may involve the mouth, throat, eye, heart, and bloodstream.

It has been proposed that many medical conditions are associated with an "overgrowth" of *Candida*, which is known as Candidiasis hypersensitivity, polysystemic candidiasis, or chronic candidiasis syndrome. *Candida* hypersensitivity has been specifically suggested to be involved in MS. It is claimed that it may occur with MS because of MS-associated immune system abnormalities or the use of steroids, which suppress the immune system. In addition to MS, candidiasis hypersensitivity has been associated with fatigue, depression, anxiety, schizophrenia, rheumatoid arthritis, AIDS, breathing problems, and bladder infections. It is claimed that 30 percent of people in United States have candidiasis hypersensitivity. Demonstrating the presence of the organism is apparently not necessary to make the diagnosis. These ideas have been popularized Drs. William Crook and Orion Truss.

Treatment Method

Several treatment measures often are recommended for people with suspected candidiasis hypersensitivity. These include avoidance of moldy environments and dietary changes to eliminate foods that might contain yeast. Therapy also may involve the use of vitamin supplements and antifungal drugs such as nystatin, ketoconazole, or amphotericin.

Studies in MS and Other Conditions

There is no evidence that *Candida* plays an important role in MS or in conditions other than obvious *Candida* infections. No large clinical studies have shown drug or diet therapy for *Candida* to be beneficial for MS or MS-associated symptoms.

Side Effects

If *Candida* therapy is considered, it must first be discussed with a physician. The antifungal drugs used for this therapy are generally well tolerated. However, they occasionally produce liver inflammation and, in rare situations, they have caused fatal liver injury.

Conclusion

Treatment for *Candida* should be approached cautiously. There is no strong evidence that *Candida* causes MS or that treatment for *Candida* improves the course of the disease or symptoms of MS. Rarely, toxicity is associated with the medications used for treatment.

Additional Readings

Journal Articles

Bennett JE. Searching for the yeast connection. *N Engl J Med* 1990;323:1766–1767.
Blonz ER. Is there an epidemic of chronic candidiasis in our midst? *JAMA* 1986;256:3138–3189.

12

Chelation Therapy

Chelation therapy is a procedure in which metal-binding chemicals are given for health reasons. This form of treatment has sometimes been claimed to be effective for multiple sclerosis (MS). It is estimated that chelation therapy is used by tens of thousands of people in the United States for MS and other health problems.

Treatment Method

In chelation therapy, ethylenediaminetetraacetic acid (EDTA) is given through an intravenous infusion. EDTA binds strongly to (chelates) harmful metals, and the metal-EDTA complexes then are excreted in the urine. Vitamin and mineral supplements are also frequently given. A course of treatment may involve 20 to 30 infusions that are given over the course of a few months. This type of therapy is effective for known situations of heavy-metal toxicity, such as lead poisoning.

Some chelation products can be taken orally. These are of no proven value, and the U.S. Food and Drug Administration (FDA) has determined that they should not be sold.

Studies in MS and Other Conditions

Chelation therapy has been recommended by some for the treatment of MS. Since 1955, some proponents have advocated its use for heart disease because it can presumably remove calcium from the harmful plaques on blood vessels. Chelation therapy also has been recommended for people with strokes, Parkinson's disease, Alzheimer's disease, muscular dystrophy, heart disease, narrowing of peripheral blood vessels (peripheral vascular disease), cancer, and arthritis.

The only clear indication for chelation therapy is heavy-metal poisoning. Limited studies have suggested a possible benefit for stroke—further studies are needed in this area. No well-designed studies support the use of chelation therapy for MS, and studies in heart disease and peripheral vascular disease have shown no clear benefit for chelation therapy.

Side Effects

Chelation therapy has potential risks. Side effects include kidney injury, bone marrow damage, anemia, breathing difficulty, irregular heart rhythms, low blood pressure, low blood levels of calcium and sugar (glucose), bleeding problems, and inflammation at the sites used for intravenous lines. Rarely, fatalities may occur. Fourteen deaths were attributed to chelation therapy in one clinic.

Practical Information

Chelation therapy is expensive. A course of treatment may cost between $3,000 and $5,000.

Conclusion

No well-documented clinical or scientific studies indicate that chelation therapy is an effective treatment for MS. Rarely, it may produce serious side effects, and it is very expensive.

Additional Readings

Books

Cassileth BR. *The Alternative Medicine Handbook*. New York: W.W. Norton, 1998, pp. 152–153, 176–178.

Ernst E, ed. *The Desktop Guide to Complementary and Alternative Medicine: An Evidence-Based Approach*. Edinburgh: Mosby, 2001, pp. 43–44.

Kowalak JP, Mills EJ, eds. *Professional Guide to Complementary and Alternative Therapies*. Springhouse, PA: Springhouse Publishing, 2001, pp. 138–140.

Navarra T. *The Encyclopedia of Complementary and Alternative Medicine*. New York: Checkmark Books. 2005, p. 26–27.

Spencer JW, Jacobs JJ. *Complementary and Alternative Medicine: An Evidence-Based Approach*. St. Louis: Mosby, 2003, pp. 156–157, 213–214.

13

Chiropractic Medicine

Chiropractic medicine is one of the most popular forms of complementary and alternative medicine (CAM) in the United States. Chiropractors are the largest group of alternative medicine practitioners and the third largest group of health care professionals in the United States (after physicians and dentists). It is estimated that more than 160 million Americans visit chiropractors yearly.

Part of the popularity of this therapy in the United States may be due to the fact that chiropractic medicine, unlike many other forms of CAM, was founded in this country. It was developed by Daniel D. Palmer, in Iowa, in the 1890s. Some form of spinal manipulation, as used in chiropractic medicine, also has been practiced in other cultures, including ancient Egypt and ancient Greece.

Chiropractic medicine has been severely criticized by mainstream medical professionals. The American Medical Association (AMA) has long questioned the effectiveness and safety of chiropractic medicine. In the 1960s, the AMA passed a resolution banning physicians from association with chiropractors and established a board, The Committee on Quackery, to discourage the use of chiropractors. In 1990, the Supreme Court ruled that the AMA was guilty of a conspiracy to "contain and eliminate" the chiropractic profession.

Treatment Method

Chiropractors believe that mild bone abnormalities of the spine are the cause of many medical disorders. According to this theory, the function of those nerves that leave the spine is altered by *subluxations* or misalignments of the bones of the spine. As a result, these bony abnormalities may produce nerve pressure, which may then affect many different muscles and organs of the body. This is sometimes compared to the decreased flow of water caused by standing on a garden hose and the increased, normal flow of water, caused by taking one's foot off the hose. Chiropractors attempt to treat these bone abnormalities through a variety of spinal manipulation techniques or *adjustments*, which presumably normalize the bone positions. In addition to this theory of spinal manipulation, chiropractic medicine holds that the body is able to heal itself; chiropractic medicine discourages the use of drugs and surgery.

Two groups of chiropractors are recognized: "straights" and "mixers." Straights use only spinal manipulation. Mixers, who represent the majority of chiropractors in the United States, use manipulation techniques and other measures, which may include ultrasound, massage, herb or vitamin supplements, and dietary recommendations.

Studies in MS and Other Conditions

No well-documented clinical trials demonstrate that chiropractic therapy improves the course of multiple sclerosis (MS) or improves MS-specific symptoms. Studies of chiropractic medicine applied to MS are limited to clinical studies with significant shortcomings or to isolated reports of individual responses to this therapy.

Musculoskeletal conditions that are seen in MS may respond favorably to chiropractic therapy. Most notably, multiple studies have evaluated the chiropractic treatment of low back pain, which may occur in people with MS. Of note, besides chiropractors, physical therapists and osteopaths also perform spinal manipulation. In addition, low back pain may resolve with no therapy at all and may respond to nonmanipulative forms of therapy given by primary care doctors, orthopedic physicians, neurologists, and physical therapists. The relative effectiveness and expense of these different approaches is debatable. In 1994, the Agency for Health care Policy and Research endorsed chiropractic therapy for low back pain that is recent and not longstanding.

The effects of chiropractic therapy on neck pain are less clear. Some studies have reported positive results, but this is less definitive than are the studies of low back pain. Also, a rare chance exists of producing a stroke through manipulation for neck pain (see "Side Effects").

Chiropractic therapy has been investigated in other conditions. Among neurologic disorders, small or single-case studies note beneficial responses in people with headaches and spinal cord injury. These studies are too small to be conclusive. Chiropractic therapy sometimes is recommended for many other conditions, including asthma, ear infections, and gastrointestinal disorders. No strong evidence supports its use in these conditions.

Side Effects

Chiropractic therapy usually is well tolerated. Only 135 complications were reported between 1900 and 1980. Most complications are from neck manipulation. For people with serious diseases or symptoms, it is important to be evaluated and treated fully by a physician and not to substitute chiropractic medicine for conventional medicine. This is because chiropractors are not as well trained in diagnosis as physicians.

For people who pursue chiropractic therapy, one of the more common adverse effects is achy muscles, which may last for 1 to 2 days after therapy. Chiropractic treatment may also cause headaches and fatigue. One significant possible complication is stroke associated with neck manipulation. This is very rare (1 in 20,000 to 1 in approximately 3,000,000), but it also may be very serious. Bone fractures and injuries to disks are also very rare. Injuries to nerves of the lower spine as a result of lower back manipulation (cauda equina syndrome) are also extremely rare.

Chiropractic manipulation should be avoided by women who are pregnant and by people with spinal-bone fractures or dislocations, spine trauma, severe disk herniations, cancer or infection of the bone, severe osteoporosis, severe arthritis, severe diabetes, and those undergoing treatment with blood-thinning medications.

Practical Information

Chiropractic treatment often is done on a weekly basis. The initial visit is 30 to 60 minutes in length and may cost from $60 to $225. Follow-up visits, which typically take 10 to 20 minutes, may cost $30 to $75. Medicare, Medicaid, and some private health insurance plans may cover the cost of chiropractic therapy.

The amount of therapy needed depends on the individual and the type of problem. The number of visits is typically two to fifteen. For low back pain, improvement typically starts within four weeks, and the entire therapy course generally lasts six to eight weeks.

Chiropractors are licensed in all states. More information about chiropractic medicine and practitioners may be obtained from:

- The American Chiropractic Association (www.amerchiro.org), 1701 Clarendon Boulevard, Arlington VA 22209 (703-276-8800 or 800-986-4636).
- International Chiropractors Association (www.chiropractic.org), 1110 North Glebe Road, Suite 650, Arlington VA 22201 (703-528-5000 or 800-423-4690).

Conclusion

There is no strong published evidence that chiropractic therapy is beneficial for MS attacks or in altering the overall course of the disease. However, low back pain, which may occur with MS, responds positively to chiropractic manipulation. There is less supportive evidence that chiropractic therapy improves neck pain and headaches. Users of chiropractic therapy should be aware of the rare side effects, including stroke, and should rely on physicians, not on chiropractors, for the diagnosis and treatment of potentially serious conditions.

Additional Readings

Books

Ernst E, ed. *The Desktop Guide to Complementary and Alternative Medicine: An Evidence-Based Approach*. Edinburgh: Mosby, 2001, pp. 45–48.

Haldeman S, Hooper P. Chiropractic approach to neurologic illness. In: Weintraub MI, Micozzi MS, eds. *Alternative and Complementary Treatment in Neurologic Illness*. New York: Churchill Livingstone. 2001, pp. 93–108.

Navarra T. *The Encyclopedia of Complementary and Alternative Medicine*. New York: Checkmark Books. 2005, pp. 27–29.

Swenson RS, Haldeman S. Chiropractic. In: Oken BS, ed. *Complementary Therapies in Neurology: an Evidence-Based Approach*. London: Parthenon Publishing Group, 2003, pp. 27–49.

Journal Articles

Elster E. Eighty-one patients with multiple sclerosis and Parkinson's disease undergoing upper cervical chiropractic care to correct vertebral subluxation: a retrospective analysis. *J Vertebral Sublux Res* 2004; August:1–9.

Ernst E. Chiropractic care: attempting a risk-benefit analysis. *Am J Public Health* 2002;92:1603–1604.

Ernst E, Harkness E. Spinal manipulation: a systematic review of sham-controlled, double-blind, randomized clinical trials. *J Pain Symptom Management* 2001; 22:879–889.

Hurwitz IL, Morganstern H, Harber P, et al. A randomized trial of medical care with and without physical therapy and chiropractic care with and without physical modalities for patients with low back pain: 6-month follow-up outcomes from the UCLA back pain study. *Spine* 2002;27:2193–2204.

Kaptchuk TJ, Eisenberg DM. Chiropractic—origins, controversies, and contributions. *Arch Intern Med* 1998;158:2215–2224.

Smith WS, Johnston SC, Skalabrin EJ, et al. Spinal manipulative therapy is an independent risk factor for vertebral artery dissection. *Neurol* 2003;60:1424–1428.

14

Colon Therapy, Detoxification, and Enemas

Colon therapy has been practiced in some form for thousands of years. It was used in ancient Egypt and ancient Greece. The use of colon therapy in the United States began in the 1890s. At that time, it was often part of the therapy provided at health spas. One of the most well-known colonic therapists was John Harvey Kellogg, who, after treating thousands of people with colon therapy, went on to found the Kellogg cereal company. The popularity of colon therapy waned during the 1940s but has grown significantly since that time. It is estimated that tens of thousands of Americans are currently treated using colon therapy. Colon therapy sometimes is suggested for people with multiple sclerois (MS) and also as a component of preventive health care.

Treatment Method

In colon therapy, the large intestine, or colon, is cleansed with liquid. Plastic tubes are placed in the rectum, and a solution, which may be water or water mixed with herbs, coffee, or enzymes, is then passed through the tubing and into the colon. The solution is eventually passed out through one of the tubes in the rectum. Although an ordinary enema generally uses about 1 quart of water, a session of colon therapy may use 20 or more gallons of water. Colon therapy sessions last approximately 1 hour.

Colon therapy is claimed to be beneficial because it involves "detoxification." It is believed that waste material on the walls of the intestine is toxic and that this material is absorbed into the bloodstream and produces disease. This toxic material is removed through colonic irrigation, and beneficial effects are allegedly produced.

Studies in MS and Other Conditions

No studies document that colon therapy is beneficial for MS. Colon therapy does not appear to be effective for any other medical condition. Standard enemas are effective for constipation.

Side Effects

It is important to be aware of possible serious side effects from colon therapy. Intestinal infections may develop if sanitary procedures are not used. In some well-known cases from the 1980s, people died from severe intestinal infections following colon therapy. Colon therapy also may produce generalized weakness, worsen hemorrhoids, cause chemical imbalances, and produce perforations, or holes, in the intestine. Colon therapy may be more dangerous in people with known diseases of the intestine, such as Crohn's disease, colon cancer, ulcerative colitis, and diverticulitis.

Conclusion

Colon therapy should be discussed with a physician. There are no documented beneficial effects for people with MS. This type of treatment also may produce serious side effects.

Additional Readings

Books

Cassileth BR. *The Alternative Medicine Handbook*. New York: W.W. Norton, 1998, pp. 179–182.

Ernst E, ed. *The Desktop Guide to Complementary and Alternative Medicine: An Evidence-Based Approach*. Edinburgh: Mosby, 2001, p. 79.

Hafner AW, Zwicky JF, Barrett S, et al. *Reader's Guide to Alternative Health Methods*. American Medical Association, 1993, pp. 293–295.

Navarra T. *The Encyclopedia of Complementary and Alternative Medicine*. New York: Checkmark Books. 2005, pp. 29–30.

15

Cooling Therapy

Cooling therapy is a unique form of complementary and alternative medicine (CAM) used for people with multiple sclerosis (MS). Small decreases in body temperature may lead to relief of some MS-related symptoms. Cooling methods ranging from the simple to the complex have been developed. The use of cooling suits for MS was introduced in the United States in the early 1990s.

The effect of heat on MS symptoms has been known for years. A worsening of symptoms with small increases in body temperature occurs in 60 to 80 percent of people with MS. In fact, the "hot bath test" was one of the earliest tests for diagnosing MS. In this test, which is no longer used, people suspected of having MS were placed in a hot bath and assessed for any worsening of symptoms. Similarly, early in the course of MS, the only noticeable manifestation of the disease may be a symptom, such as weakness, numbness, or visual blurring, that occurs only in situations that increase body temperature, such as exercise, sunbathing, fever, or warm showers or baths.

Although warming may produce a worsening of symptoms, cooling may lead to improvement. This cooling effect has been observed with cold baths or exposure to cold air, both of which may produce short-term decreases in the severity of MS-associated symptoms. This beneficial response to cooling is the basis of cooling therapy.

Unlike some forms of CAM, cooling therapy has a scientific basis. Nerve cells that have damage to the insulating part of the cell (the myelin), as occurs in MS, exhibit a blocked conduction of signals with small increases in temperature. Thus, small decreases in temperature may facilitate transmission of nerve signals.

Treatment Method

Different techniques may be used to elicit cooling. Simple measures include taking cool showers or baths, sitting near a fan or air conditioner, using an ice pack, wearing cotton clothing, avoiding warm environments, and drinking cold liquids. More sophisticated approaches utilize a garment, such as a vest, that produces body cooling. Cooling garments may be "passive" or "active." Passive garments, which use ice packs or evaporation for cooling, are simpler and more portable than are active garments. Coolants actively circulate through active garments, which appears to result in more effective cooling.

Studies in MS and Other Conditions

Small research studies indicate that cooling produces improvement in MS symptoms. One of the older studies, reported in the late 1950s, showed that a temperature reduction of as little as 1° Fahrenheit led to noticeable benefits. A 1995 investigation of six people with MS showed that cooling primarily improved fatigue and leg strength (1). In a 1999 Swedish study of 10 people with MS, cooling suits relieved multiple symptoms (2). Beneficial effects included improvement in walking, transferring, and urinating. Overall, an increased ability of people to care for themselves was noted. Results in other studies indicate cooling-associated improvement in fatigue, spasticity, visual changes, speech difficulties, sexual disorders, cognition, tremor, and coordination.

At the Rocky Mountain Multiple Sclerosis Center, we conducted a survey of heat sensitivity and cooling strategies in more than 2,500 people with MS. We found that the most common heat-related symptoms were fatigue and weakness. The most commonly used methods of cooling were air conditioning, fans, and ice packs. A relatively small fraction of people had tried cooling garments—17 percent had used passive cooling garments, while 4 percent had tried active cooling garments. For both types of garments, the most common symptoms that improved were fatigue and weakness. The garments were generally well tolerated. The most common negative comments for both types of garments were that they were cumbersome and looked unusual. The complete results of this survey are available at the CAM website of the Rocky Mountain Multiple Sclerosis Center (www.ms-cam.org).

A rigorous study of cooling in MS was reported in 2003 (3). In this relatively large study, 84 people with MS and heat sensitivity were evaluated for both the short- and long-term effects of cooling. The cooling apparatus used in this research involved technology developed at the National Aeronautics and Space Administration (NASA). For the short-term component of the study, low-dose and high-dose cooling were administered for 1 hour. For the group that received high-dose cooling, a small amount of improvement was noted in multiple objectively measured parameters, including walking speed and visual abilities. Less notable changes were observed with low-dose cooling. In the long-term portion of the study, the effects of daily cooling over 1 month were examined. By self assessment, people believed they improved in fatigue, strength, and thinking processes during this time.

Side Effects

In general, the use of cooling garments is well tolerated. There may be a feeling of discomfort when cooling begins. Some people report that handling the garments is cumbersome.

It is important to keep in mind that individual variation occurs in the amount of cooling and the extent of benefit. Some people exhibit little or no reduction in body temperature with cooling. In approximately 10 percent of people with MS, a *paradoxical response* may occur, and symptoms may actually worsen with cooling therapy.

Practical Information

Cooling garments are available from several sources and are manufactured by:

- Akemi, Inc. (www.bodycooler.com), 8700 Commerce Park Drive, Suite 212, Houston TX 77036 (800-209-2665)
- Cool-Sport (www.coolsport.net), 2008 West Carson Street, Suite 211, Torrance CA 90501-3297 (310-618-1590)
- CoolSystems, Inc. (www.rechargems.com), 929 Camelia Street, Berkeley CA 94710 (510-559-3940)
- Jenkins Comfort Systems (www.jenkinscomfort.com), P.O. Box 10063, Augusta GA 30903 (888-508-6908)
- Life Enhancement Technologies, Inc. (www.2bcool.com), 807 Aldo Avenue, Suite 101, Santa Clara CA 95054 (800-779-6953)
- Maverick Marketing Ventures, Inc. (www.soothsoft.com/chillow.htm), P.O. Box 38159, Colorado Springs CO 80937-8159 (888-244-5569)
- MicroClimate Systems, Inc. (www.microclimate.com), 965 East Saginaw Road, Sanford MI 48657 (800-397-3004)
- Polar Products, Inc. (www.polarsoftice.com), 540 South Main Street, Suite 951, Akron OH 44311 (800-763-8423)

- Shafer Enterprises, L.L.C. (www.coolshirt.net), 10 Andrew Drive, Suite 200, Stockbridge GA 30281 (800-345-3176)
- Steele Incorporated (www.steelevest.com), P.O. Box 7304, Kingston WA 98346 (888-783-3538)

Health insurance coverage for cooling garments may be available.

Conclusion

Limited research studies have found that cooling produces improvement in multiple MS-associated symptoms, including weakness, fatigue, spasticity, walking difficulties, urinary difficulties, speech disorders, visual difficulties, sexual problems, incoordination, tremor, and cognitive difficulties. This therapy is usually well tolerated. Cooling therapy may make the transition from unconventional to conventional medicine in the future.

Additional Readings

Journal Articles

Brenakker EA, Oparina TI, Hartgring A, et al. Cooling garment treatment in MS: clinical improvement and decrease in leukocyte NO production. *Neurol* 2001;57:892–894.

Capell E, Gardella M, Leandri M, et al. Lowering body temperature with a cooling suit as symptomatic treatment for thermosensitive multiple sclerosis patients. *Ital J Neurol Sci* 1995;16:533–539.

Feys P, Helsen W, Liu X, et al. Effect of peripheral cooling on intention tremor in multiple sclerosis. *J Neurol Neurosurg Psych* 2005;76:373–379.

Flensner G, Lindencrona C. The cooling-suit: a study of ten multiple sclerosis patients' experience in daily life. *J Adv Nursing* 1999;29:1444–1453.

Guthrie TC, Nelson DA. Influence of temperature changes on multiple sclerosis: critical review of mechanisms and research potential. *J Neurol Sci* 1995; 29:1–8.

Ku Y-T, Montgomery LD, Lee HC, et al. Physiologic and functional responses of MS patients to body cooling. *Am J Phys Med Rehabil* 2000;79:427–434.

Ku Y-T, Montgomery LD, Webbon BW. Hemodynamic and thermal responses to head and neck cooling in men and women. *Am J Phys Med Rehab* 1996; 75:443–450.

Ku YT, Montgomery LD, Wenzel KC, et al. Physiologic and thermal responses of male and female patients with multiple sclerosis to head and neck cooling. *Am J Phys Med Rehab* 1999;8:447–456.

NASA/MS Cooling Study Group. A randomized controlled study of the acute and chronic effects of cooling therapy for MS. *Neurol* 2003;60:1955–1960.

16

Craniosacral Therapy

Craniosacral therapy, also known as cranial therapy, cranial osteopathy, and craniopathy, is a form of bone manipulation derived from chiropractic and osteopathic medicine. Dr. William G. Sutherland initially developed the technique in the United States in the early 1900s. A modified version was developed by Dr. John Upledger in the 1970s. Dr. Upledger currently provides instruction in this therapy to large numbers of health care providers through the Upledger Institute in Florida.

Treatment Method

Craniosacral therapy focuses on the bones of the skull, spine, and pelvis. Through massage, craniosacral therapy presumably facilitates the smooth flow of the cerebral spinal fluid, a watery liquid that surrounds the brain and spinal cord. According to the theory, more freely flowing cerebral spinal fluid results in improved functioning of the central nervous system, immune system, and other bodily processes. Craniosacral therapists claim that they can detect the rhythmic movements of the skull bones.

Studies in MS and Other Conditions

The basic ideas that underlie craniosacral therapy are not consistent with the conventional understanding of skeletal anatomy or nervous-system functioning. There is no evidence that demonstrates that impaired cerebral spinal fluid flow is a common cause of disease or that craniosacral massage significantly alters cerebral spinal fluid flow. Also, it is not clear that craniosacral therapy rhythm is a meaningful measurement or that it can be reliably detected.

In addition to the lack of scientific rationale for craniosacral therapy, there is a paucity of clinical research. Craniosacral therapy has not been specifically investigated in multiple sclerosis (MS). Dr. Upledger writes: "We have treated a large number of multiple sclerosis patients with only moderate success. We often find a rather significant emotional component along with multiple sclerosis. Most often the emotional resistance is such that we have been unable to achieve optimal results with craniosacral therapy" (1).

Beneficial effects are claimed for many disorders, including brain injury, spinal cord injury, pain, and seizures. However, these claims usually are based on the experiences of individuals (anecdotes) rather than on formal clinical trials.

Craniosacral therapy should be avoided in infants and children because the skull bones are not stable at a young age and manipulation could produce injury. Adverse effects of craniosacral therapy have been described in adults. Mild headaches were reported in one study of 55 people with mild head injury (2). In addition, three people, or approximately 5 percent, reported more serious side effects. These included dizziness and body stiffness (spasticity), both of which may be present in MS. Craniosacral therapy should be avoided by those with brain aneurysms (outpouching of blood vessels in the brain), bleeding in the brain, and increased pressure within the brain (increased intracranial pressure). Practitioners of craniosacral therapy state that the therapy may increase the effects of psychiatric, epileptic, and diabetic medications.

Practical Information

Craniosacral therapy sessions generally last from 30 to 60 minutes and cost between $50 and $250. For short-term conditions, one to three sessions over 1 to 3 weeks may be recommended. Longer-term conditions may require weekly treatment for several months. The number of treatment sessions needed varies. Therapy may be performed by chiropractors, osteopaths, naturopaths, physical therapists, nurses, massage therapists, and physicians.

Conclusion

Most claims about craniosacral therapy are not supported by clinical studies. Side effects may occur in 5 percent of people treated. The theoretical basis for the therapy is not consistent with the current understanding of the nervous system.

Additional Readings

Books

Cassileth BR. *The Alternative Medicine Handbook*. New York: W.W. Norton, 1998, pp. 222–225.

Ernst E, ed. *The Desktop Guide to Complementary and Alternative Medicine: An Evidence-Based Approach*. Edinburgh: Mosby, 2001, pp. 48–50.

Navarra T. *The Encyclopedia of Complementary and Alternative Medicine*. New York: Checkmark Books. 2005, p. 31.

Upledger JE. *Craniosacral Therapy*. Berkeley, CA: North Atlantic Books, 2001.

Journal Articles

Green C, Martin CW, Bassett K, et al. A systematic review of craniosacral therapy: biological plausibility, assessment reliability and clinical effectiveness. *Compl Ther Med* 1999;7:201–207.

Greenman PE, McPartland JM. Cranial findings and iatrogenesis from craniosacral manipulation in patients with traumatic brain syndrome. *J Am Osteopath Assoc* 1995;95:182–188, 191–192.

Hanten WP, Dawson DD, Iwata M, et al. Craniosacral rhythm: reliability and relationships with cardiac and respiratory rates. *J Orthoped Sports Phys Ther* 1998;27:213–218.

Moran RW, Gibbons P. Intraexaminer and interexaminer reliability for palpation of the cranial rhythmic impulse at the head and sacrum. *J Manipulative Physiol Ther* 2001;24:183–190.

Rogers JS, Witt PL, Gross MT, et al. Simultaneous palpation for the cranialsacral rate at the head and feet: intrarater and interrater reliability and rate comparisons. *Phys Ther* 1998;78:1175–1185.

17

Dental Amalgam Removal

The removal of dental amalgam has been proposed as a therapy for multiple sclerosis (MS). This treatment is based on the idea that metal is slowly released from amalgam and causes or worsens MS.

Dental amalgam is composed of mercury as well as silver, copper, tin, and zinc. Amalgam has been used for more than 150 years to fill cavities and is used currently for 80 to 90 percent of tooth restorations.

Very small amounts of mercury are released from amalgam in teeth in the form of solid mercury and mercury vapor. It is claimed that the mercury released from amalgam damages the immune system and nervous system and thereby causes MS and other diseases. In addition, it has been proposed that disease is caused by harmful allergic reactions to the mercury or to the electrical currents generated by mercury. The presumed mercury toxicity is termed *mercury hypersensitivity, mercury sensitivity, mercury toxicity,* and *micromercurialism.* Electricity generated by mercury is called *electrogalvinism* or *oral galvanism.*

Treatment Method

A specific procedure often is followed when amalgam removal is considered. Questionnaires about symptoms may be administered. The evaluation may include electrical readings of restorations, skin-patch allergy testing, mercury-vapor tests, and hair analysis. Amalgam removal may be done by removing a few fillings at a time; this technique is claimed to release "locked mercury." Gold or plastic fillings are used after amalgam removal.

Studies in MS and Other Conditions

Dental amalgam has been implicated in MS on the basis of several claims and observations. Anecdotal reports exist of people with MS benefiting from amalgam removal. Also, MS has been associated with both dental caries—the bacterial disease of teeth that produces cavities—and dental treatment. Finally, it has been proposed that MS is caused by exposure to mercury or other heavy metals.

Dental amalgam has been implicated in many other diseases. These include diseases that may have an immunologic basis, such as arthritis, lupus, and chronic fatigue syndrome, as well as other neurologic diseases, such as headache, epilepsy, brain tumor, and Parkinson's disease. Amalgam also has been implicated in depression, cancer, and heart disease.

Contrary to what sometimes is claimed, no evidence demonstrates that mercury causes MS or that the removal of dental amalgam improves the course of MS. Although mercury toxicity may produce symptoms that resemble those of MS, the underlying pathologic processes of mercury toxicity are quite different from those of MS. The levels of mercury in the brain are similar for people with MS and the general population. In addition, some people with MS have no dental amalgam, and MS was recognized as a disease before amalgam was used routinely in dental practice. Some studies of large populations have shown a trend for people with MS to have more dental caries than the general population—these trends, however, have not been statistically significant. Finally, the amount of mercury released from amalgam is very low. Studies in the early 1980s first indicated that relatively high levels of mercury are released, but subsequent studies demonstrated low levels of mercury release.

It is estimated that mercury from amalgam constitutes 10 percent or less of all the mercury consumed by an individual; other sources of mercury are food (especially fish), pollution, medications, paints, and disinfectants. For dental amalgam to produce mercury levels that are associated with even minimal toxic effects, it has been calculated that an individual would need approximately 500 amalgam surfaces or approximately 200 dental fillings.

Although some anecdotal reports document benefit from amalgam removal, no well-designed studies demonstrate that dental amalgam removal improves the course of MS. Studies of large numbers of people with MS have not shown any association between dental treatment and MS attacks. Dentists and dental staffs are exposed to relatively high doses of mercury and have blood mercury levels that are three to five times higher than the general population, yet MS is no more common in the dental profession than in the general population.

Professional guidelines do not recommend amalgam removal for MS. The medical advisory board of the National Multiple Sclerosis Society of the United States, the Public Health Service, and the National Institutes of

Health (NIH) do not support this treatment. In 1987, the American Dental Association (ADA) determined that unnecessary amalgam removal is improper and unethical. In 1996, a Colorado dentist who actively performed amalgam removal on people with MS had his dentist's license revoked by the Colorado State Board of Medical Examiners.

No evidence demonstrates that significant allergies to mercury cause disease. Allergy to mercury actually is very rare and, when it does occur, it produces swelling of the tissues around an amalgam-filled tooth; it has not been associated with other diseases.

No large, well-documented studies have formally evaluated this treatment. In other words, no large group of people with MS has been studied to determine if removing amalgam produces a statistically better clinical course than not removing amalgam. Although the ideal clinical study has not been conducted, it is not clear that enough suggestive evidence warrants the time, resources, and expense of such a study.

Side Effects

In general, dental amalgam removal is well tolerated. Rarely, it can damage nerves or tooth structure. For a short time, removal of amalgam may actually increase blood levels of mercury.

Conclusion

It is very difficult to determine with absolute certainty whether a compound such as dental amalgam is completely safe. The ideal clinical studies in MS have not been conducted. However, based on available evidence, there is no strong indication that dental amalgam removal has a beneficial effect on MS. Amalgam removal is usually well tolerated, but it may be very expensive.

Additional Readings

Journal Articles

Bates MN, Fawcett J, Garrett N, et al. Health effects of dental amalgam exposure: a retrospective cohort study. *Int J Epidemiol* 2004;33:1–9.

Casetta I, Invernizzi M, Granieri E. Multiple sclerosis and dental amalgam: case-control study in Ferrara, Italy. *Neuroepidemiology* 2001;20:134–137.

Ekstrand J, Bjorkman L, Edlund C, et al. Toxicological aspects on the release and systemic uptake of mercury from dental amalgam. *Eur J Oral Sci* 1998; 106:678–686.

Eley BM, Cox SW. The release, absorption, and possible health effects of mercury from dental amalgam: a review of recent findings. *Brit Dental J* 1993; 175:355–362.

Fung YK, Meade AG, Rack EP, et al. Brain mercury in neurodegenerative disorders. *J Toxicol Clin Toxicol* 1997;35:49–54.

Mackert JR, Berglund A. Mercury exposure from dental amalgam fillings: absorbed dose and the potential for adverse health effects. *Crit Rev Oral Biol Med* 1997; 8:410–436.

NIH Conference Assessment. Effects and side-effects of dental restorative materials. *Adv Dental Res* 1992;6:1–144.

Sheridan P. Amalgam restorations and multiple sclerosis. *MS Management* 1997;4:21–40.

18

Diets and Fatty-Acid Supplements

A possible role of diet in multiple sclerosis (MS) was proposed more than 50 years ago. Since that time, this area has been a source of much controversy and confusion. Issues related to diet may be especially confusing for people with MS because some diet advocates exaggerate claims, and many health care professionals do not discuss the topic in much depth or with much enthusiasm.

A Well-Balanced Diet

It is essential to appreciate the basic components of a healthy diet before considering details about the possible influence of diet on MS. Regardless of an individual's specific diet, adequate amounts of a variety of foods should be consumed. Previously, the U.S. Department of Agriculture (USDA) provided general guidelines for food intake in the form of a pyramid. In 2005, the Food Guide Pyramid was replaced by MyPyramid, an approach that emphasizes a more individualized approach to diet and lifestyle. Guidelines are based on one's age, sex, and physical activity level. Recommendations are provided for the intake of grains, vegetables, fruits, dairy, meat/beans, and oils. MyPyramid can be accessed through a website, www.mypyramid.gov.

The MyPyramid system is based on the *2005 Dietary Guidelines for Americans*, which was released by the USDA and the U.S. Department of Health and Human Services in January 2005. The following are some of these guidelines:

- Consume a variety of nutrient-dense foods and beverages.
- Limit the intake of saturated and trans fats, cholesterol, added sugars, salt, and alcohol.
- Participate in regular physical activity.

87

- Consume adequate amounts of fruits and vegetables.
- Eat a variety of vegetables and fruits each day.
- Consume three or more ounces of whole-grain products daily.
- Consume less than 10 percent of calories from saturated fats.
- Maintain total fat intake to between 20 and 35 percent of calories.
- Consume fiber-rich foods.
- Limit sodium intake.

Two Therapies versus One Therapy

Diets and fatty-acid supplements may affect MS by interacting with the immune system. Conventional medications for MS (Copaxone, Avonex, Betaseron, Rebif, Novantrone, Tysabri) also interact with the immune system. It is not known whether combining one of these conventional medications with a dietary approach would be beneficial. Because we have a limited understanding of the regulation of the immune system, it is conceivable, although unlikely, that a combination could be harmful. If a single approach is chosen, far more convincing evidence exists for one of the conventional medications than for a dietary approach.

Dietary Fat

A possible association of MS with dietary fat has been proposed. In the body, fats, which are stored in fatty tissue, are important for producing energy and providing the necessary chemical structure for the outer surfaces or membranes of all cells in the body. Fats are made up of *fatty acids*, long chains of carbon atoms attached to each other. Hydrogen and oxygen atoms are attached to these chains.

Two types of fats exist. One is *saturated fat*, which is hard at room temperature and is what we generally think of as "fat." The fat on meat is one of the most important forms of this type of fat. Saturated fat also is present in butter and hard cheese. The fatty acids in saturated fats will not allow any more hydrogen atoms to attach to them. In other words, the fatty acids are already "saturated" with hydrogen.

Another type of fat is *unsaturated fat* or unsaturated fatty acids. Unsaturated fat is soft or liquid at room temperature and is frequently referred to as "oil." Examples of unsaturated fat include margarine and oils from vegetables, seeds, and fish.

The fatty acids in unsaturated fats exist in two forms. *Monounsaturated fatty acids*, which are present in olive oil, have one position at which hydrogen atoms may attach. *Polyunsaturated fatty acids* have two or more positions at which hydrogen atoms may attach. The body is not able to make polyunsaturated fatty acids. As a result, polyunsaturated fatty acids are essential in the diet and are referred to as *essential fatty acids.*

Polyunsaturated fatty acids have been the subject of most dietary studies in MS. Two important forms of polyunsaturated fatty acids exist. One type is known as *omega-six* (or ω-6), a term that relates to the chemical structure of these fatty acids. Different forms of omega-six fatty acids exist, and these different forms may be converted into each other by a pathway of chemical reactions (Figure 18.1).

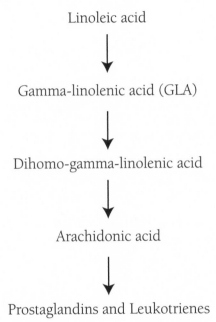

Linoleic acid

↓

Gamma-linolenic acid (GLA)

↓

Dihomo-gamma-linolenic acid

↓

Arachidonic acid

↓

Prostaglandins and Leukotrienes

FIGURE 18.1. *Biochemical pathway of omega-six fatty acids.*

The first fatty acid in the omega-six pathway is *linoleic acid.* Linoleic acid is present in a variety of foods, especially the oils of seeds and nuts. It is converted to gamma-linolenic acid (GLA). GLA is not nearly as common in food as linoleic acid. Relatively high levels of GLA are only present in unusual sources such as evening primrose oil. Further chemical reactions convert GLA to dihomo-gamma-linolenic acid and then to arachidonic acid. Finally, arachidonic acid is converted to prostaglandins and other chemicals that may be important for regulating the immune system and other body processes.

The other important polyunsaturated fatty acid is known as omega-three (or ω-3) fatty acid. Fish and other seafood are the most well-known sources of this fatty acid. Once again, there is a pathway of different omega-three fatty acids (Figure 18.2). The first fatty acid in this pathway is alpha-linolenic acid, which is present in green leafy vegetables and flaxseed (or linseed) oil. Alpha-linolenic acid is then converted to eicosapentaenoic acid (EPA) and docosa-hexanoic acid (DHA). Both of these fatty acids are present in fish and fish oils. DHA is converted to prostaglandins and leukotrienes, which are the same types of chemicals found at the end of the omega-six pathway.

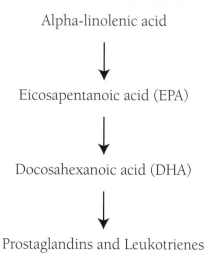

FIGURE 18.2.   *Biochemical pathway of omega-three fatty acids.*

MS and Polyunsaturated Fatty Acids

For years, MS has been associated with polyunsaturated fatty acids. In the early 1950s, studies were conducted in several countries to evaluate the possible impact of food intake on MS. Some of these studies suggested that MS was more common in areas where the consumption of saturated fat, especially animal fat, was relatively high. Some research also associated MS with a high intake of dairy products. In contrast, in some studies, populations with a relatively high intake of polyunsaturated fatty acids, including vegetable oil and fish, appeared to have lower rates of MS.

As a result of the studies of polyunsaturated fatty acids in the diet of different populations, the actual levels of polyunsaturated fatty acids were determined in people with MS. Some, but not all, blood studies found decreased levels of polyunsaturated fatty acids, especially omega-six fatty acids such as linoleic acid. A few studies also reported decreased levels of omega-three fatty acids.

Many hypotheses have been proposed for the possibly decreased polyunsaturated fatty-acid levels in MS. One hypothesis is that people with MS have some type of abnormality in the fatty-acid chemical pathway. Another hypothesis is that people with MS do not eat adequate amounts of polyunsaturated fatty acids.

How could fatty acids have anything to do with MS? When the original fatty-acid studies were conducted, it was claimed that people with MS may have blood that is too thick and, as a result, flows slowly or "sludges." This idea is not consistent with our current scientific understanding of MS. It also has been proposed that, because polyunsaturated fatty acids are an important component of the lining of nerve cells (myelin), an abnormality of polyunsaturated fatty acids could produce abnormalities in the myelin, as is observed in MS. A more current idea is that prostaglandins and other chemicals in the pathway of the omega-six and omega-three fatty acids (Figures 18.1 and 18.2) decrease the activity of the immune system. This immune-suppressing effect may be beneficial because the immune system is excessively active in MS.

Fats and Other Diseases

The effect of dietary fat on diseases other than MS also has been examined. Saturated fat, especially animal fat, increases cholesterol levels, and high cholesterol levels are associated with heart disease and stroke. In addition, some studies have associated high blood pressure and some forms of cancer with a high intake of saturated fats. Consequently, a diet relatively low in saturated fat and relatively high in polyunsaturated fat has general health benefits.

Specific Diets

The Swank Diet

Some of the original studies on MS and dietary fat were done by Dr. Roy Swank. Because of the apparent association of dietary fat with MS, in 1948, he began treating people with MS with a specific diet. The diet involves a very low intake of saturated fat and a high intake of polyunsaturated fatty acids. Saturated fat is decreased to 15 grams per day. No red meat is allowed in the first year. Thereafter, 3 ounces of red meat per week are permitted. The diet does not allow high-fat dairy products or processed foods that contain saturated fats. A high intake of polyunsaturated fatty acids, cod liver oil supplements, frequent meals with fish, and a multivitamin also is recommended.

In 1970, Dr. Swank reported the results of his diet in people with MS (1). On average, he observed patients over a 17-year period. People on the diet had less frequent and less severe attacks, less worsening of their overall neurologic condition, and a decreased death rate. The diet was reported to be most beneficial when it was started in people who were early in the disease course or who had mild disability. Some of the results were dramatic. For example, he described a 95 percent reduction in the frequency of MS attacks.

A follow-up report was published in 1990 (2). In this report, 144 patients were monitored over 34 years. Once again, the diet produced significant benefits and appeared to be especially effective when started in people who were mildly affected or were early in the disease course.

In 2003, Dr. Swank published another follow-up to his initial clinical trial (3). This report described people who had been on his diet for 50 years. Of the 15 people who were examined, only two had significant disability. The other 13 people had done well neurologically, had "joyful laughter," and "appeared youthful." Although these findings are impressive, no description of standard neurologic test results was given, and the examined group represented only a small subgroup of the 144 people who were originally enrolled in the study.

As noted, this diet is strict. Saturated fat intake is very low and polyunsaturated fat intake is high. Because of the decreased intake of meat, people who follow this diet should be certain that protein intake is adequate.

Most physicians and other health care professionals have a reserved approach to the Swank diet because the study was not carried out by guidelines that are now traditionally used in trials of new medical therapies. In particular, patients were not randomly given a specific therapy (randomization), the clinician who examined the patients was aware of their treatment (in other words, the clinician was not "blinded"), and no placebo-treated group was used.

The Swank diet is a fairly extreme dietary approach without strong clinical studies to support its use. More details and specific recipes are provided in a book by Dr. Swank and Barbara Dugan, *The Multiple Sclerosis Diet Book*.

Other Low-Fat Diets

Other low-fat diets are more conservative than the Swank diet. It is not clear that the Swank diet is superior to these other low-fat diets; no clinical studies have compared the Swank diet with a less strict low-fat diet. General dietary guidelines that decrease saturated fats, increase fiber and polyunsaturated fatty acids, and maintain a well-balanced diet are outlined in Table 18.1. These guidelines are relatively easy to follow, are practical, and may produce beneficial effects.

TABLE 18.1. *General Diet Guidelines That May Be of Benefit for MS and General Health*

- Eat a variety of foods.
- Choose whole grain cereals and breads.
- Eat several daily servings of fruits and vegetables.
- Decrease total fat in diet to 30 percent or less of calories.
- Limit saturated fat intake.
- Eat fish two to three times per week.
- Choose a diet moderate in salt, sugar, and alcoholic beverages.
- Drink plenty of fluids and water.

The dietary recommendations in Table 18.1 have not been tested clinically. However, it could be beneficial for people with MS and may improve general health by decreasing the risk of heart disease, stroke, and possibly other conditions.

Other Dietary Considerations in MS

Constipation is a frequent complaint in people with MS. One way to improve constipation is to increase the amount of fiber in the diet. Good sources of fiber include whole grain breads and cereals, as well as fruits and vegetables. An increased intake of water and other fluids also may be beneficial for constipation; six to eight 8-oz. glasses of fluid daily generally are recommended. Some people with MS may have frequent urinary tract infections, and increased fluid intake also may be helpful for this problem. Finally, for some people with MS-associated fatigue, it may be beneficial to avoid large increases or decreases in the blood sugar level. This may be accomplished by eating small meals and snacks throughout the day.

Several other dietary factors should be kept in mind. Alcohol may, over the short-term, produce or worsen fatigue, bladder problems, walking difficulty, or clumsiness in the arms and legs. Grapefruit juice may increase the effects of many medications, including some that are commonly used for MS—diazepam (Valium), clonazepam (Klonopin), carbamazepine (Tegretol), sildenafil (Viagra), and sertraline (Zoloft).

Many diets have been recommended for MS with little or no supportive evidence. Avoiding foods that may cause allergies has been suggested. One example of this approach is a diet that does not contain gluten, a major component of wheat and wheat products. One clinical trial of a gluten-free diet in MS found no benefit, and a study of the animal model of MS found that a gluten-free diet actually *worsened* the disease. Studies of the blood and intestinal lining of people with MS do not indicate a sensitivity to gluten. No evidence supports the use of a pectin-free diet or a severely sugar-restricted diet.

If a specific diet is followed, it is important to always maintain a well-balanced intake of nutrients. Some of the more extreme dietary approaches that focus on one specific aspect of the diet may actually create problems by causing nutrient deficiencies.

Supplements of Polyunsaturated Fatty Acids

In addition to modifying the diet, the intake of polyunsaturated fatty acids may be increased by taking supplements. Some of these supplements actually have been studied in clinical trials of people with MS.

Omega-Six Polyunsaturated Fatty Acids

Linoleic Acid

Studies of Linoleic Acid. Supplementation with linoleic acid, the first chemical in the omega-six fatty-acid pathway (see Figure 18.1), has been extensively studied. In EAE, an animal model of MS, supplements of linoleic acid are beneficial, whereas deficiencies of linoleic acid are harmful.

Three studies have been undertaken of linoleic acid supplements in people with relapsing MS. Linoleic acid was given as some form of sunflower seed oil in these studies. All three studies meet the formal clinical research criteria of being randomized, blinded, and placebo-controlled.

The first study was reported in 1973 (4). Seventy-five people were studied over 2 years, and the daily dose of linoleic acid was 17.2 grams. Treatment produced decreased duration and severity of attacks. No effect was noted on the frequency of attacks or the progression of the disease.

The second study was published in 1978 (5). Over a 2-year period, 116 people were studied. As in the first study, the severity and duration of attacks were significantly improved, but there was no change in the frequency of attacks or the progression of disability.

The third study also was reported in 1978 (6). Seventy-six people with MS were monitored over 2.5 years. In contrast to the two other studies, no benefit was found in this investigation.

In summary, two studies produced limited positive results and one study found no benefit. To attempt to clarify the mixed results of these studies, a combined analysis was published in 1984 (7). The information on a total of 172 people from all three studies was pooled. It was noted that, in the third study, which did not report any benefit, the people had more severe MS and had MS for a longer time than did people in the other two studies. Using the combined analysis, linoleic acid treatment slowed the progression of disability in people with little or no disability at the start of the treatment. Regardless of the duration or severity of the disease, linoleic acid treatment was associated with reduced length and severity of attacks. The statistical methods used in this combined analysis have been questioned. Overall, the effects of linoleic acid supplements on MS are suggestive but not definitive.

Sources of Linoleic Acid.   Good sources of linoleic acid are the oils of seeds and nuts, such as safflower oil, sunflower oil, and sesame seed oil. Flaxseed (or linseed) oil contains linoleic acid as well as omega-three fatty acids (see section on omega-three fatty acids). Seeds and nuts themselves also contain linoleic acid.

A simple measure to increase linoleic acid intake is to increase the consumption of linoleic acid-containing foods, including oils. A more aggressive approach is to take oil supplements. The optimal dosage of linoleic acid is not known. In addition, the amount of omega-six fatty acids relative to the amount of omega-three fatty acids (the omega-six:omega-three ratio) is probably important, but the most desirable ratio of these fatty acids has not been established.

It is sometimes recommended that approximately 4 teaspoons of linoleic acid–containing oils be taken daily. The oil may be used in salad dressings or mixed in with vegetables, yogurt, or soft cheese. It should not be heated and should be stored under cool and dark conditions.

Risks of Linoleic Acid.   The most significant concern that has been raised about this type of supplementation is that it may increase the risk of cancer. This concern is based primarily on studies in animals. A 1998 review of all animal and human studies in this area of research concluded that it was unlikely that linoleic acid supplementation increased the risk of several types of cancer in humans. This issue has not yet been fully resolved.

Other issues are important to consider with linoleic acid supplementation. The oily taste may be unpleasant, and diarrhea may occur in some people. Omega-6 fatty-acid supplements may increase triglyceride levels in those with elevated triglyceride levels. Polyunsaturated fatty acids in general may produce vitamin E deficiency; low doses of vitamin E supplements may be indicated (see the next section). The possible adverse effects of long-term supplementation have not been studied formally and consequently are not known.

Gamma-Linolenic Acid (GLA)

Studies of GLA.   Evening primrose oil is a popular supplement sometimes recommended for MS because it contains GLA, which is one step beyond linoleic acid in the omega-six biochemical pathway (see Figure 18.1).

There are some theoretical reasons why GLA may be better than linoleic acid, but scant clinical information exists in this area. A preparation of evening primrose oil (Naudicelle) was used in one of the linoleic acid trials in 1978. Eight capsules daily were not effective. In the same trial, linoleic acid alone was somewhat beneficial for relapsing MS. It should be noted that low doses of GLA (340 milligrams daily) were used in this trial, and it is possible that higher doses could have produced a benefit. However, this would have meant consuming up to 40 evening primrose oil capsules daily!

Two other limited studies have been undertaken of evening primrose oil in relapsing MS. One of these studies also used a drug known as *colchicine*. Both studies produced some positive results. However, they involved a small number of people and did not include a placebo-treated group. Consequently, it is difficult to be confident about the results. A 1977 study of people with progressive MS found no benefit for evening primrose oil (8).

Scientific studies indicate that GLA suppresses immune system activity. In rats, evening primrose oil decreases the activity of *T cells*, a type of immune cell. GLA supplementation decreases the severity of disease in mice and rats with EAE, an animal model of MS.

Evening primrose oil has been claimed to be effective for many other conditions. Conflicting results have been obtained in studies of other immune diseases, such as rheumatoid arthritis. Evening primrose oil may decrease breast pain (mastalgia), increase bone density in those with osteoporosis, and be helpful for two skin conditions — eczema and atopic dermatitis.

In summary, the limited clinical information about GLA supplementation in MS does not strongly support its use. However, only low doses have been studied clinically, and scientific studies and clinical studies in other diseases suggest that it may be effective. In theory, GLA could provide the same benefits as linoleic acid, but high doses may be necessary, and such high doses may not be practical on a regular basis because of its cost.

Sources of GLA.   Very few sources of GLA exist. Evening primrose oil is one of the most commonly recommended sources. It contains 8 to 10 percent GLA and approximately 70 percent linoleic acid. A single evening primrose oil capsule generally contains about 40 milligrams of GLA. Some capsules of evening primrose oil also contain vitamin E in low levels, such as 10 international units (IU) per capsule.

An Australian study evaluated the consistency of evening primrose oil preparations (9). Fourteen of 16 different preparations contained reasonable amounts (7 to 10 percent) of GLA. Because of the presence of other fatty acids in some of the capsules, it was proposed that borage seed oil, another source of GLA, may have been added to these preparations.

If evening primrose oil is taken, approximately six capsules daily are often recommended. It should be kept in mind that GLA is present in low levels; six capsules daily result in a daily dose of only approximately 240 milligrams. As a result, other omega-six fatty acids (see the earlier sections) may need to be taken as well if one is attempting to significantly increase the total intake of omega-six fatty acids.

GLA is found in several other sources. *Borage seed oil*, which is sometimes recommended, is a rich source of GLA. It contains 20 to 26 percent GLA, more than twice the amount in evening primrose oil. However, borage seed oil may contain chemicals (pyrrolizidine alkaloids) that are toxic to the liver. As a result, it is safest to avoid borage seed oil. Some borage seed oil preparations claim to be free of pyrrolizidine alkaloids.

Like borage seed oil, black currant seed oil contains a higher concentration of GLA (14 to 19 percent) than does evening primrose oil. However, this oil has not been well studied with regard to possible toxic chemicals or adverse effects. *Spirulina*, or blue-green algae, may contain high concentrations of GLA, but the amount of GLA in a given spirulina product usually is not specified and may be negligible (see "Herbs"). Finally, one of the more obscure sources of GLA is human breast milk.

In conclusion, evening primrose oil generally is preferred over other products for supplementation with GLA. Borage seed oil, black currant seed oil, and spirulina are of uncertain safety or contain variable and uncertain amounts of GLA.

Risks of GLA.   In general, evening primrose oil is well tolerated. Long-term human studies indicate that a daily dose up to 2,800 milligrams of GLA is not generally associated with any serious side effects.

Some concerns arise with the use of evening primrose oil and other sources of GLA. Because sources of GLA usually contain linoleic acid, the adverse effects and risks of linoleic acid are present. These include an unpleasant taste and soft stools or diarrhea. Additional concerns with evening primrose oil include the expense, as well as nausea and headache. Evening primrose oil and borage seed oil may provoke seizures in people taking antipsychotic medications. Evening primrose oil may affect blood clotting. Therefore, it probably should be avoided by people who take blood-thinning medications or high doses of aspirin, people who have blood-clotting disorders, and people who are undergoing surgery. The safety of black currant seed oil and Spirulina are not known, and borage seed oil may contain liver toxins.

All supplements containing polyunsaturated fatty acids may produce vitamin E deficiency. Consequently, low doses of vitamin E supplements should be taken if vitamin E is not already present in the fatty-acid supplement.

Omega-Three Fatty Acids

Studies.   One large study has been undertaken of omega-three fatty-acid supplement use in MS (10). This 2-year study, reported in 1989, involved 312 people and daily treatment with 10 grams of fish oil. The daily doses of specific fatty acids were 1.7 grams of EPA and 1.1 grams of DHA (see Figure 18.2). People in this study also were instructed to increase omega-six fatty-acid intake and to decrease animal fat intake. In the untreated group, 52 percent worsened, whereas in the treated group, 43 percent worsened. A trend was noted toward a beneficial effect, but formal analysis showed that this effect was not quite statistically significant.

A small 1986 study evaluated the effect of cod-liver oil supplements, which contain omega-three fatty acids, on the MS attack rate in 10 people with MS (11). A beneficial effect of treatment was noted, but this study is limited by several factors, including the absence of a placebo-treated group and treatment that involved vitamin D, calcium, and magnesium in addition to cod-liver oil.

Another study of 16 people with MS evaluated the effects of omega-3 fatty-acid supplements, other dietary supplements (vitamins A, B, C, D, and E), and dietary advice (including decreased saturated fat and increased fish intake) over 2 years (12). Compared with clinical status before the study, treatment was associated with a significant decrease in the attack rate and improvement in the level of disability. No placebo group was used in this small study.

A study of 31 people with MS assessed the effects of omega-3 fatty-acid supplements in combination with glatiramer acetate (Copaxone) or interferons (Avonex, Betaseron, Rebif) (13). People were treated with the conventional MS medications along with either fish oil and a very low-fat diet or with olive oil and a low-fat diet. A trend for improved emotional and physical functioning was found in those taking fish oil—these results were not statistically significant. Both dietary approaches were associated with a decrease in attack rate.

Other scientific and clinical aspects of omega-three fatty acids are under active investigation. Studies of immunologic function indicate that, in laboratory animals and in humans, omega-three fatty-acid supplementation decreases the activity of several components of the immune system. In limited studies of EAE, omega-three fatty acids have produced variable effects. Some studies actually indicate that omega-three fatty acids worsen the disease, but others indicate beneficial effects.

Studies of immune diseases other than MS have indicated a possible therapeutic effect with the use of omega-three fatty acids. Omega-three fatty-acid supplements appear to decrease joint stiffness and joint swelling in rheumatoid arthritis. These supplements may be helpful for another immune condition known as *antiphospholipid antibody syndrome.*

Omega-three fatty acids may have other important health benefits. They have the potential to prevent and treat heart disease. They appear to decrease blood levels of triglycerides and mildly decrease blood pressure.

Sources of Omega-Three Fatty Acids.   Fish is a common food source of omega-three fatty acids. Thus, a simple approach to increase omega-three fatty-acid intake is to increase the consumption of fish, especially fatty fish such as salmon, Atlantic herring, Atlantic mackerel, bluefin tuna, sardine, and cod liver. Two to three servings of fish weekly are sometimes recommended. A very high intake of fish raises concerns about mercury toxicity, especially among women who are pregnant or may become pregnant. Fish with relatively high mercury levels include shark, swordfish, and king mackerel.

Omega-three fatty acids also may be consumed as supplements. The optimal dose of omega-three fatty acids is not known. Also, the amount of omega-three fatty acids relative to that of omega-six fatty acids (omega-six:omega-three ratio) may be important, but currently not enough information is known to make specific recommendations.

Fish oil and cod liver oil supplements are available as liquid oil or as capsules. Concentrated EPA and DHA also are available. Multiple fish oil products have been analyzed and have not been found to contain any detectable mercury. Total daily doses of 3 grams or less are believed to be safe. One tablespoon of fish oil contains approximately 140 calories and 14 grams of fat.

A unique source of omega-three fatty acids is flaxseed (or linseed) oil, which contains both omega-three and omega-six fatty acids. The omega-three fatty acids are in the form of alpha-linolenic acid (see Figure 18.2), as opposed to EPA and DHA, which are present in fish oil and cod-liver oil. Of note, alpha-linolenic acid may not produce as potent effects as do EPA and DHA. (Interestingly, walnuts are also a source of alpha-linolenic acid.) Linoleic acid is the omega-six fatty acids in flaxseed oil. Consuming flaxseed oil is a way to obtain both omega-three and omega-six fatty acids from a single source. One tablespoon of flaxseed oil daily sometimes is recommended.

Risks of Omega-Three Fatty Acids.   In 1997, the U.S. Food and Drug Administration (FDA) determined that fish oil supplements were generally safe when the total daily intake of EPA and DHA was less than 3 grams. In one long-term study of 295 people, no serious adverse effects were observed with 7 years of fish oil use.

Cod-liver oil has a fishy taste, and flaxseed oil has a bitter taste; these unpleasant tastes may be lessened by cooling the oils. Daily doses greater than 45 grams of flaxseed oil may have a laxative effect, and daily doses greater than 60 grams may theoretically increase blood levels of cyanide-containing compounds. Vitamin E deficiency may potentially develop when taking omega-three fatty acids; supplemental vitamin E should be taken.

Most commercial fish oil products do not contain vitamin A. However, halibut, shark, and cod-liver oils contain relatively high levels of vitamin A. Excessive doses of these oils should be avoided, because high levels of vitamin A may be toxic, especially during pregnancy (see "Vitamins, Minerals, and Other Nonherbal Supplements").

Omega-three fatty-acid supplements impair lung function in those with aspirin sensitivity. These supplements also may increase blood sugar levels in diabetic patients and produce excessive mental and physical activity, a condition known as *hypomania*, in people with depression or manic-depressive illness, It is not known if omega-three fatty-acid supplements are safe in women who are pregnant or breast-feeding.

Finally, fish oils, specifically EPA, may inhibit blood clotting. These oils should be used with caution by people who are undergoing surgery, people who have blood-clotting disorders, and people who take blood-thinning medication or high doses of aspirin.

Vitamin E and Polyunsaturated Fatty Acids

Polyunsaturated fatty acids may decrease vitamin E levels. As a result, if high levels of polyunsaturated fatty acids are consumed in the diet or through the use of supplements, vitamin E intake must be increased. However, *high doses* of vitamin E do not appear to be necessary. According to many recommendations, the ratio of vitamin E (in international units, or IU) to polyunsaturated fatty acids (in grams) should be 0.6 to 0.9. This means that, on a daily basis, 0.6 to 0.9 IU of vitamin E are needed for each gram of polyunsaturated fatty acids. Consequently, given an intake of 25 grams of polyunsaturated fatty acids, only 15 to 22 IU of vitamin E would be required. It is sometimes stated that hundreds of IU of supplemental vitamin E are needed if polyunsaturated fatty-acid supplements are taken. This does not appear to be true. In fact, because it may be best to avoid high doses of vitamin E and other antioxidants in MS, as discussed elsewhere in the section on vitamins, lower doses of vitamin E, such as 100 IU may be adequate and may actually be more appropriate. Some omega-three fatty-acid supplements, such as evening primrose oil capsules, contain vitamin E, in which case additional vitamin E may not be necessary.

Other Supplements Sometimes Recommended with Polyunsaturated Fatty Acids

In addition to vitamin E, several other supplements sometimes are recommended with the use of polyunsaturated fatty acids. Vitamin B_6 (pyridoxine) and zinc are recommended by some because the fatty-acid chemical pathway uses vitamin B_6 and zinc. In fact, the intake of these micronutrients from the diet is probably adequate and, in the case of zinc, supplements pose a theoretic risk because they may stimulate the immune system (see "Vitamins, Minerals, and Other Nonherbal Supplements"). If these supplements are taken, the daily dose of vitamin B_6 should not exceed 50 milligrams, and low doses of zinc should be taken (see "Vitamins, Minerals, and Other Nonherbal Supplements").

For antioxidant supplementation, vitamin C and beta-carotene sometimes are recommended in addition to vitamin E. As noted, only low doses of additional vitamin E appear to be needed, and there is no strong evidence that additional antioxidant vitamins are required. Because the benefits and risks of antioxidant vitamins in MS are not known, as discussed in the section on vitamins, it is not clear that vitamin C and beta-carotene supplements are beneficial. In fact, it is possible that, in higher doses, they may be immune-stimulating and therefore may negatively affect the course of MS. If vitamin C and beta-carotene supplements are used, they probably should be taken in moderation (see "Vitamins, Minerals, and Other Nonherbal Supplements").

In summary, low doses of supplemental vitamin E may be required when high levels of polyunsaturated fatty acids are consumed. It is not clear that a need exists for any other supplements, including vitamin B_6, zinc, vitamin C, and beta-carotene.

Conclusion

Different Interpretations of Information

The area of diets and fatty-acid supplementation in MS is controversial. This review of the positive and negative evidence shows that some suggestive studies exist, especially those with omega-six fatty acids. However, these studies are not definitive.

With the information available, it is striking how many different interpretations and recommendations one can find. Some vendors of supplements and some books on CAM are overly enthusiastic about dietary changes, discuss only the positive results, and recommend diet changes and supplements for all people with MS.

On the other hand, more conservative conclusions and recommendations are made in the conventional medical literature. However, even within mainstream medicine, a spectrum of interpretations may be found:

■ In an American text, *Merritt's Textbook of Neurology*, it is stated: "Diet therapy and vitamin supplements are frequently advocated, but no special supplementation or elimination diet has proved to be more beneficial than a well-balanced diet…" (14).

■ In a textbook on MS, Dr. Donald Paty, a Canadian neurologist who conducted the negative study of linoleic acid, states: "…perhaps [linoleic acid] should be reinvestigated in MS… one cannot object to or condone such self-therapy… one can understand the patient's desire to take a preparation that is not harmful if it might possibly have a beneficial effect" (15).

■ A text by a Swiss physician, Dr. Jurg Kesselring, is more specific: "[The diet] can be enriched with cold-pressed oils which are rich in essential fatty acids… vitamin E supplements are to be recommended… capsules can provide, at best, a supplement to the essential fatty acids in the diet" (16).

■ In a 1989 medical journal article, Dr. David Bates, who conducted several of the fatty-acid trials, comments: "[T]here does appear to be a genuine, though mild, improvement with supplements of the diet by both omega-six and omega-three polyunsaturated fatty acids" (17).

Different Approaches

What is the correct approach in this area? Why are there so many different opinions? Much of the confusion and controversy in this area is due to a difference in perspective. Overall, there probably is no single correct approach. However, within a given perspective, there may well be a correct approach.

From a conservative, mainstream perspective, one would state that the results are not definitive and that no recommendations can be made until further studies are done. A more aggressive and unconventional approach is to state that the results are suggestive and that, because changing the diet and using supplements is probably not harmful, there may be some benefit to dietary changes and supplement use. These different approaches are outlined below.

■ *Conventional Approach.* Because the study results are not conclusive at this time, a conventional approach would involve no dietary changes or possibly modest alterations in the diet. No supplements would be recommended. This approach often is taken by physicians and other health care professionals and can be summarized as:

- Diet—No modifications or modified as in Table 18.1
- Supplements—None

■ *Unconventional Approach—Moderate*. Because of the suggestive results of the research studies, this approach involves some dietary changes and supplement use. This is an approach sometimes taken by people with MS who would like to make dietary changes and feel an urgency to act on study results that are suggestive but not definitive. This approach is:

- Diet—Modified as in Table 18.1
- Supplements:
  - Omega-six—moderate amounts of sunflower seed (or other) oil and possibly evening primrose oil
  - Omega-three—moderate amounts of a supplement such as fish oil; cod-liver oil and flaxseed oil are other options but may be less desirable than fish oil
  - Vitamin E—Modest doses as indicated

■ *Unconventional Approach—Aggressive*. This approach involves a significant change in diet as well as high-level supplementation. It generally is not recommended by health care professionals, but sometimes is used by people who want to pursue all measures that decrease saturated fat intake and increase polyunsaturated fatty-acid intake:

- Diet—Swank diet or similar diet
- Supplements:
  - As in Swank diet, also evening primrose oil
  - Vitamin E—As indicated

A Final Cautionary Word

Several important factors must be kept in mind when considering any diet or fatty-acid supplement use in MS. First, the prescription medications for MS (Copaxone, Betaseron, Avonex, Rebif, Novantrone, and Tysabri) are proven and effective therapies; diet or supplement use is not. *Changes in diet or supplement use should not be used in lieu of taking these conventional medications.*

Additionally, if diets or supplements are used in addition to the conventional medications, it is important to recognize that the effects of this combination therapy are not known. Presumably, two different approaches would be better than one, but the immune system and MS are not fully understood. It is conceivable, although unlikely, that a combination treatment such as this might be less beneficial than using conventional medicine alone.

Additional Readings

Books

Bowling AC, Stewart TS. *Dietary Supplements and Multiple Sclerosis: A Health Professional's Guide*. New York: Demos Medical Publishing, 2004.

Fragakis AS. *The Health Professional's Guide to Popular Dietary Supplements*. The American Dietetic Association, 2003.

Jellin JM, Batz F, Hitchens K. *Natural Medicines Comprehensive Database*. Stockton, CA: Therapeutic Research Faculty, 2005.

Polman CH, Thompson AJ, Murray TJ, Bowling AC, Noseworthy JH. *Multiple Sclerosis: The Guide to Treatment and Management*. New York: Demos Medical Publishing, 2006.

Swank RL, Dugan BB. *The Multiple Sclerosis Diet Book*. New York: Doubleday, 1987.

Ulbricht CE, Basch EM, eds. *Natural Standard Herb and Supplement Reference: Evidence-Based Clinical Reviews*. St. Louis: Elsevier-Mosby, 2005.

Journal Articles

Anon. Omega-3 oil: fish or pills? *Consumer Reports* 2003;July:30–32.

Bates D, Cartlidge NEF, French JM, et al. A double-blind controlled trial of long chain n-3 polyunsaturated fatty acids in the treatment of multiple sclerosis. *J Neurol Neurosurg Psychiatry* 1989;52:18–22.

Bates D, Fawcett PRW, Shaw DA, et al. Polyunsaturated fatty acids in treatment of acute remitting multiple sclerosis. *Br Med J* 1978;2:1390–1391.

Bates D, Fawcett PRW, Shaw DA, et al. Trial of polyunsaturated fatty acids in non-relapsing multiple sclerosis. *Br Med J* 1977;10:932–933.

Bowling AC, Stewart TM. Current complementary and alternative therapies of multiple sclerosis. *Curr Treat Opt Neurol* 2003; :55–68.

Calder PC. Fat chance of immunomodulation. *Trends Immunol Today* 1998; 19:244–247.

Dworkin RH, Bates D, Millar JHD, et al. Linoleic acid and multiple sclerosis: a reanalysis of three double-blind trials. *Neurology* 1984;34:1441–1445.

Horrobin DF. Multiple sclerosis: the rational basis for treatment with colchicine and evening primrose oil. *Med Hyp* 1979;5:365–378.

Lauer K. Diet and multiple sclerosis. *Neurology* 1997;49:S55–S61.

Manley P. Diet in multiple sclerosis. *Practitioner* 1994;238.

Meyer-Reinecker HJ, Jenssen HL, Kohler H, et al. Effect of gamma-linoleate in multiple sclerosis. *Lancet* 1976;10:966.

Miller JHD, Zilkha KJ, Langman MJS, et al. Double-blind trial of linoleate supplementation of the diet in multiple sclerosis. *Br Med J* 1973;1:765–768.

Nordvik I, Myhr KM, Nyland H, et al. Effects of dietary advice and Ω-3 supplementation in newly diagnosed MS patients. *Acta Neurol Scand* 2000;102:143–149.

Paty DW, Cousin HK, Read S, et al. Linoleic acid in multiple sclerosis: failure to show any therapeutic benefit. *Acta Neurol Scand*, 1978;58:53–58.

Stewart TM, Bowling AC. Polyunsaturated fatty acid supplementation in MS. *Int MS J* 2005;12:88–93.

Swank RL. Multiple sclerosis: twenty years on low fat diet. *Arch Neurol* 1970;23:460–474.

Swank RL, Dugan BB. Effect of low saturated fat diet in early and late cases of multiple sclerosis. *Lancet* 1990;336:37–39.

Swank RL, Goodwin J. Review of MS patient survival on a Swank low saturated fat diet. *Nutrition* 2003;16:161–162.

Weinstock-Guttman, Baier M, Park Y, et al. Low fat dietary intervention with omega-3 fatty acid supplementation in multiple sclerosis patients. *Prostaglandins Leukotrienes Essential Fatty Acids* 2005;73:392–404.

19

Enzyme Therapy

Enzymes are a type of protein used by the body to perform chemical reactions. Enzymes break down food in the digestive tract and carry out essential chemical functions in the rest of the body. It is claimed that treatment with enzymes is beneficial for many diseases, including multiple sclerosis (MS).

Enzyme therapy has a long history. In one form of possible enzyme therapy, the Indians of Central America and South America traditionally use the leaves and fruit of papaya trees and the fruit of pineapples to treat inflammatory conditions. John Beard, a Scottish embryologist, first used enzyme therapy for cancer treatment in 1902. During the 1920s, Dr. Edward Howell claimed that consuming large amounts of enzymes was a way to help the body not deplete its own natural enzyme supply. In Germany, during the 1960s and 1970s, enzyme treatment was recommended for MS, cancer, viral infections, and a variety of inflammatory conditions. Enzyme therapy was promoted by Drs. Max Wolf and Karl Ransberger.

Two major types of enzyme therapy are used. In *digestive enzyme* therapy, advocates claim that digestive enzyme supplements improve the breakdown of food, increase nutrient absorption, and decrease the accumulation of toxins. Through these mechanisms, enzyme therapy is believed to effectively treat hundreds of diseases and maintain health. In the other type of enzyme therapy, *systemic enzyme therapy*, it is believed that special enzyme preparations pass through the stomach undigested and then are absorbed into the bloodstream from the intestines. Whether this process occurs, and whether it offers any benefit, is unproven. It is claimed that enzyme therapy has been used by many well-known public figures, including Charlie Chaplin, Marlene Dietrich, J. Edgar Hoover, Aldous Huxley, members of the Kennedy family, Marilyn Monroe, and Pablo Picasso.

Enzyme therapy was under much scrutiny in the United States during the 1980s. In 1986, the U.S. Food and Drug Administration (FDA) ordered one company, Enzymatic Therapy, Inc., to discontinue its published research bulletins because of false claims. Subsequently, the FDA continued to monitor informational seminars and material produced by the company. In 1992, the use of false claims by the company was prohibited by a court order.

Treatment Method

Most enzyme therapy involves taking supplements that contain enzymes obtained from animals or plants. Digestive enzymes from animal sources include proteases (chymotrypsin and trypsin), amylases, and lipases. Examples of plant-derived enzymes are bromelain from pineapples, papain from papaya, and ficin from figs. In Europe, intravenous infusions of enzymes or enemas of enzyme-containing solutions also sometimes are recommended.

Rare situations occur in which enzyme therapy is used in conventional medicine. These conditions include pancreatitis, cystic fibrosis, and Gaucher disease. An enzyme known as *lactase* is given for people who cannot tolerate dairy products (lactose-intolerance). People with excessive gas may find relief from Beano, an enzyme (alpha-galactosidase) that improves the digestion of high-fiber foods, such as beans, peas, and whole grains.

Studies in MS

Specific enzyme treatment regimens, along with vitamin and mineral supplements, are sometimes recommended for people with MS. Surprisingly, some of these enzymes and other supplements are suggested because they stimulate the immune system. Despite the detailed and lengthy recommendations offered for MS, no clinical research evidence supports this therapy.

A form of enzyme treatment known as *oral hydrolytic enzyme therapy* has been studied in MS. Some early reports in the German medical literature suggested that this type of enzyme therapy may be helpful for MS. Also, this therapy was reported to be beneficial in the animal model of MS and to produce immune-system changes in humans that, in theory, would be beneficial for MS. Due to these observations, a study of oral hydrolytic enzyme therapy was conducted (1). This 2-year study, which included more than 300 people with relapsing MS at 22 MS clinics in Europe, compared the clinical and magnetic resonance imaging (MRI) effects of an enzyme therapy (bromelain, trypsin, rutoside) with placebo. This study met the criteria for a well-conducted clinical trial—it involved multiple clinics (*multicenter*), placebo treatment (*placebo-controlled*), the random assignment of enzyme treatment or placebo to patients (*randomized*), and patients and clinicians who were unaware of who received enzyme therapy or placebo (*double-blinded*). Unfortunately, enzyme therapy did not produce therapeutic effects on the basis of progression of disability, number of attacks, or multiple MRI criteria.

Intravenous enzyme therapy also has been proposed for MS and other immune system diseases. It is claimed that intravenous enzymes may help break down harmful "immune complexes." A preliminary study in Austria reported some beneficial effects for this therapy in MS. Enzyme-containing enemas also have been recommended for MS, but no research evidence supports their use.

Side Effects

Oral enzyme therapy is generally well tolerated. There may be changes in the color, consistency, and odor of the stools when starting treatment. Excessive gas, nausea, diarrhea, and minor allergic reactions also may occur. Ulcers may be worsened by the use of one class of enzymes known as proteases. People with hypersensitivity to pork may not tolerate pork-derived pancreatic enzymes. No significant side effects were reported in the large study of enzyme therapy in MS (1). The safety of long-term enzyme therapy has not been investigated. There is a theoretical possibility that long-term use could decrease the ability of the digestive system to secrete its own enzymes. Enzyme therapy should be avoided by women who are pregnant or breast-feeding; people who take blood-thinning medications; and people who have blood-clotting disorders, severe kidney disease, protein allergies, and recent surgical procedures. With intravenous enzyme therapy, rare but serious adverse effects are possible, including infections and severe allergic reactions.

Conclusion

In the medical literature published in English, no well-documented benefits of enzyme therapy have been noted for people with MS. A well-designed European clinical trial did not demonstrate any therapeutic effects of enzyme therapy in MS. Claims about this therapy may be exaggerated. The long-term safety of enzyme therapy has not been determined. Intravenous enzyme therapy may produce rare, but serious, side effects.

Additional Readings

Books

Cassileth BR. *The Alternative Medicine Handbook*. New York: W.W. Norton & Company, Inc., 1998:183–185.

Kowalak JP, Mills EJ, eds. *Professional Guide to Complementary and Alternative Therapies*. Springhouse, PA: Springhouse Publishing, 2001, pp. 193–194.

Journal Articles

Baumhackl U, Kappos L, Radue EW, et al. A randomized, double-blind, placebo-controlled study of oral hydrolytic enzymes in relapsing multiple sclerosis. *Mult Scler* 2005;11:166–168.

Desser L, Rehberger A, Kokron E. Cytokine synthesis in human peripheral blood mononuclear cells after oral administration of polyenzyme preparations. *Oncol* 1993;50:403–407.

Taragoni OS, Tary-Lehmann M, Lehmann PV. Prevention of murine EAE by oral hydrolytic enzyme treatment. *J Autoimmunol* 1999;12:191–198.

20

Exercise

Exercise is not always classified as a form of complementary and alternative medicine (CAM). Instead, it may be viewed as conventional medicine or entirely out of the realm of medicine, as a type of self-care or simply a component of one's lifestyle. Regardless of its formal classification, it is important to consider exercise because it is not always fully discussed during a conventional medical office visit, and it has significant health implications for people with multiple sclerosis (MS).

Attitudes about exercise and MS have changed dramatically. In the past, regular exercise was not generally recommended for people with MS. However, based on more recent research demonstrating that exercise produces multiple beneficial effects, appropriate forms of regular exercise are now encouraged for people with MS.

Treatment Method

Many possible exercise programs are possible for people with MS. They may include stretching exercises, walking, running, and a range of other exercises that may be appropriate for all levels of physical functioning. Hydrotherapy, or aquatic therapy, refers to exercising in water. This form of exercise is especially well-suited for some people with MS because water eliminates the risk of injuries from falling, and cool water may prevent body warming while exercising. In addition, exercise may be obtained by using unconventional approaches, such as yoga and t'ai chi, both of which are discussed elsewhere in this book.

The best specific type of exercise program depends on the individual. Each person with MS has specific strengths and weaknesses, and these must be taken into account when developing an exercise program. An exercise program for a person with MS is usually developed by a physical therapist.

Studies in MS and Other Conditions

Exercise may produce a wide variety of health benefits. One well-known study conducted at the University of Utah was reported in 1996 (1). In 54 people with MS, 40 minutes of aerobic exercise was done three times weekly for 15 weeks. Exercise produced benefits for physical and mental symptoms, including:

■   Weakness
■   Impaired bowel and bladder function
■   Fatigue
■   Depression
■   Anger

Similar findings have been reported in other studies. Other MS symptoms that may improve with exercise include fatigue, walking ability, and overall level of disability. Stretching exercises may decrease muscle stiffness (spasticity).

Although exercise in general may be beneficial for bladder and bowel function, a specific type of exercise called *Kegel exercises* or pelvic-floor muscle exercises may be especially helpful. With these exercises, the pelvic muscles that are used to voluntarily stop urination are flexed on a regular basis. It often is recommended that these muscles be exercised 60 to 80 times daily.

Although mixed results have been obtained, some studies show that Kegel exercises improve urinary function in both women and men by decreasing incontinence, urgency, and frequency. In some of these studies, the exercises have been combined with electrical stimulation or biofeedback (see "Biofeedback").

Men with MS may experience erection difficulties. Research indicates that pelvic exercises may improve erectile dysfunction. However, this approach is not appropriate for men with MS, because the beneficial effect occurs with erection difficulties that are due to blood flow abnormalities (venogenic erectile dysfunction), not for erection problems associated with nerve injury (neurogenic erectile dysfunction).

Studies in MS and other conditions demonstrate that exercise produces emotional benefits. In fact, more than 1,000 studies of variable quality have been conducted in the area of exercise and depression. One study that analyzed the results of 80 different clinical trials of exercise and depression found that the benefits of exercise occurred across a wide range of ages, in both sexes, and with all types of exercise. In general, longer courses of exercise (more than 17 weeks) are more effective than are shorter courses. For treating depression, exercise appears to be as effective as psychotherapy and more effective than relaxation methods or pursuing enjoyable activities. Exercise in addition to psychotherapy is more effective than exercise alone.

Although anxiety has not been studied as extensively as depression, many studies have found that exercise reduces the level of anxiety. Many different types of exercise appear to be effective for depression, and longer exercise programs (more than 10 to 15 weeks) appear to be most effective. Surprisingly, individual exercise sessions that are only 5 minutes in length appear to decrease anxiety levels. Perhaps through these effects on anxiety, a regular exercise program also may improve insomnia.

Exercise has multiple actions on the immune system. The effect that these immune system changes might have on MS has not been studied. Moderate levels of exercise have been associated with immune system activation and a decreased risk of viral infections, although strenuous exercise appears to produce mild immune suppression and an increased risk of viral infections. Because exercise has so many clear beneficial effects, the possible immune-system changes associated with exercise should not factor strongly into decision-making about exercise.

Other benefits are associated with exercise. Regular exercise may prevent *osteoporosis*, a decrease in bone density that may occur in MS. Low back pain, which also may occur in MS, may be reduced through the use of an exercise program. Large studies have found that exercise decreases the death rate by 25 to 30 percent. This may be due to the protective effect that exercise has on heart disease and stroke. Exercise may also mildly decrease blood pressure, help prevent diabetes, decrease the risk of some forms of cancer, and improve symptoms of premenstrual syndrome.

Given the many emotional and physical benefits associated with regular exercise, it is possible that a lack of exercise, or *physical deconditioning*, actually may contribute to MS-associated symptoms. Physical inactivity may worsen a wide variety of symptoms, whereas moderate levels of exercise may alleviate multiple symptoms.

An exciting area of exercise research involves proteins known as *growth factors*. A variety of these growth factors occur in the central nervous system; these usually are referred to by acronyms such as BDNF (brain-derived neurotrophic factor) and NGF (nerve growth factor). Animal studies demonstrate that regular exercise increases the brain levels of several growth factors. Growth factors have multiple effects that could be therapeutic for MS:

■   Anti-inflammatory effects: May decrease the risk of inflammation-related MS attacks

- Nerve-protecting effects: May decrease the risk of injury to nerve fibers (*axonal injury*)
- Nerve-regenerating effects: May help injured nerves grow new nerve fibers

Much of the exercise-growth factor research has focused on aging-related neurodegenerative diseases, such as Parkinson's disease, Alzheimer's disease, and Lou Gehrig's disease (amyotrophic lateral sclerosis or ALS). Exercise decreases the severity of disease in the animal models of Parkinson's disease and Lou Gehrig's disease. In addition, exercise may decrease the risk of developing Parkinson's disease. Limited studies in MS indicate that exercise may increase growth-factor levels in people with MS.

An important issue is whether exercise could improve the overall disease course of MS. It is possible that the exercise-induced increases in growth factor levels could, like the injectable MS medications, have disease-modifying effects in MS. Further research is needed to determine if exercise has such an effect.

Side Effects

The risks of exercise depend on the type of exercise. Increased body temperature associated with exercise may provoke neurologic symptoms in some people with MS. Musculoskeletal pain or injury may occur with overuse or trauma. The risk of exercise-induced injury is greater in those who are overweight, are older, or have had previous injuries. Finally, asthma may be provoked by exercise.

Practical Information

People with MS should develop an exercise program with the guidance of a physical therapist. This is especially important for those with significant physical disabilities or heart or lung conditions. Although information on exercise is readily available from popular books and recreation centers, this information should not be used instead of consulting with a professional.

Conclusion

Exercise is a simple, safe, low-cost approach that may produce many health benefits. In addition to its positive effects on general health, exercise may have a variety of beneficial effects on MS-associated symptoms, including weakness, walking difficulties, muscle stiffness (spasticity), osteoporosis, low back pain, bladder difficulties, bowel problems, fatigue, insomnia, depression, anxiety, and anger.

Additional Readings

Books

Ernst E, ed. *The Desktop Guide to Complementary and Alternative Medicine: An Evidence-Based Approach.* Edinburgh: Mosby, 2001.

Fugh-Berman A. *Alternative Medicine: What Works.* Baltimore: Williams & Wilkins, 1997: 94–100.

Journal Articles

Adlard PA, Perreau VM, Engesser-Cesar C, et al. The time course of induction of brain-derived neurotrophic factor mRNA and protein in the rat hippocampus following voluntary exercise. *Neurosci Lett* 2004;363:43–48.

Brown TR, Kraft GH. Exercise and rehabilitation for individuals with multiple sclerosis. *Phys Med Rehab Clin N Am* 2005;16:513–555.

Chen H, Zhang SM, Schwarzschild MA, et al. Physical activity and the risk of Parkinson disease. *Neurology* 2005;64:664–669.

Ernst E, Rand JI, Stevinson C. Complementary therapies for depression: An overview. *Arch Gen Psych* 1998;55:1026–1032.

Karpatkin HI. Multiple sclerosis and exercise: a review of the evidence. *Int J MS Care* 2005;7:36–41.

Petajan JH, Gappmaier E, White AT, et al. Impact of aerobic training on fitness and quality of life in multiple sclerosis. *Ann Neurol* 1996;39:432–441.

Rietberg MB, Brooks D, Uitdehaag BM, et al. Exercise therapy for multiple sclerosis. *Cochrane Database Syst Rev* 2005;1:CD003980.

Romberg A, Virtanen A, Ruutiainen J, et al. Effects of a 6-month exercise program on patients with multiple sclerosis: a randomized study. *Neurology* 2004;63:2034–2038.

Scully D, Kremer J, Meade MM, et al. Physical exercise and psychological well being: a critical review. *Br J Sports Med* 1998;32:111–120.

Solari A, Filippini G, Gasco P, et al. Physical rehabilitation has a positive effect on disability in multiple sclerosis patients. *Neurology* 1999;52:57–62.

21

Feldenkrais

Feldenkrais is a type of *bodywork* that focuses on efficient and comfortable body movements. It was developed by Moshé Feldenkrais, a Russian-born physicist. Feldenkrais is claimed to decrease stress, relieve pain, and improve balance and coordination.

Treatment Method

Very structured body movements are used in Feldenkrais. The position of the head is of particular importance. Feldenkrais usually is initially learned with lessons known as Awareness Through Movement (ATM), in which attention is focused on the motion of specific body parts during simple movements, such as walking or bending. In another type of Feldenkrais, Functional Integration (FI), more efficient movements are developed by a teacher who manipulates one's joints and muscles during movement. It is possible for people with significant disabilities to do Feldenkrais.

Studies in MS and Other Conditions

Extremely limited studies have formally evaluated Feldenkrais therapy. In a small study in multiple sclerosis (MS) conducted at the University of North Carolina, 20 people with MS received Feldenkrais or a "sham" therapy for eight weeks (1). Some of the participants had significant walking difficulties and required the use of a cane or walker. Feldenkrais did not improve arm function, multiple MS symptoms, or overall level of function. It decreased stress and may have reduced anxiety.

Feldenkrais has undergone limited study in other conditions. Preliminary studies indicate that Feldenkrais may increase neck flexibility.

Side Effects

Feldenkrais generally is regarded as a safe therapy.

Practical Information

The cost of Feldenkrais depends on the type of therapy. ATM classes cost $15 to $30, whereas FI sessions are $60 to $90. Feldenkrais usually is not covered by insurance. However, insurance coverage may be available if Feldenkrais is provided by a physical therapist or occupational therapist.

Feldenkrais may be offered at local health clubs and recreation centers. More information and a list of certified practitioners may be obtained from: The Feldenkrais Guild of North America (www.feldenkrais.com), 3611 SW Hood Avenue, Suite 100, Portland, Oregon, 97239 (800-775-2118 or 503-221-6612).

Conclusion

In summary, Feldenkrais is a safe, low- to moderate-cost therapy that has undergone limited investigation. One small study in MS indicated that Feldenkrais decreased stress and possibly reduced anxiety. Further studies are needed to determine whether it has clear beneficial effects for stress and anxiety or for other symptoms, including pain, balance, and coordination.

Additional Readings

Books

Kowalak JP, Mills EJ, eds. *Professional Guide to Complementary and Alternative Therapies*. Springhouse, PA: Springhouse Publishing, 2001, pp. 203–205.

Journal Articles

Johnson SK, Frederick J, Kaufman M, et al. A controlled investigation of bodywork in multiple sclerosis. *J Alt Complem Med* 1999;5:237–243.

22

Guided Imagery

Guided imagery is a technique frequently used in hypnosis as well as in meditation and other relaxation therapies. Although it generally is used to produce relaxation, guided imagery may be used for other purposes.

Treatment Method

In guided imagery, an individual creates images that have specific effects on the mind and body. For example, to produce a state of relaxation, one may imagine sitting in a tranquil location such as a beach or a mountain. These images may be visual but may also involve sounds, taste, and smells associated with a particular setting.

Studies in MS and Other Conditions

Guided imagery has not undergone extensive investigation in multiple sclerosis (MS). One study conducted in Pennsylvania evaluated the effects of imagery and relaxation techniques in 33 people with MS (1). For imagery, people were instructed to imagine the repair of injured myelin and beneficial immune system activity. People who practiced daily imagery along with relaxation experienced less anxiety and produced more active and powerful images of their disease process. No effect of imagery and relaxation was noted on depression or specific MS-associated symptoms. Studies in other conditions indicate that imagery may improve anxiety and pain, including cancer-related pain, postoperative pain, and headache.

Imagery could conceivably be used to alter immune system function. Limited studies in this area have produced mixed results. In one study, people were instructed to use imagery to increase the adherence, or stickiness, of *neutrophils*, a specific type of immune cell (2). Each individual created his or her own image of neutrophil adherence. For example, one person envisioned ping-pong balls that exuded honey onto their surfaces and thereby adhered to all objects that they touched. The stickiness of the neutrophils increased in one of the groups that practiced imagery.

Guided imagery has been used for other conditions. Imagery is sometimes used to assist in managing heart disease because of its relaxation effect and ability to decrease blood pressure. Elite athletes use imagery to enhance athletic performance.

Side Effects

Imagery generally is well tolerated. It should not be used instead of conventional medication for serious conditions, such as modifying the course of MS. People with psychiatric conditions, including severe depression, should use caution with imagery. Also, imagery-induced relaxation may cause disturbing thoughts, fear of losing control, and anxiety.

Practical Information

Most imagery sessions last 20 to 30 minutes. Books and audiotapes are available for additional instruction. Alternatively, a trained therapist may be used. More information about guided imagery may be obtained from: The Academy of Guided Imagery (www.academyforguidedimagery.com), 30765 Pacific Coast Highway, Suite 369, Malibu, California 90265 (800-726-2070).

Conclusion

Guided imagery is inexpensive and safe. It may reduce anxiety and pain, but its therapeutic effects have not been fully investigated. Further studies are needed to examine its effectiveness.

Additional Readings

Books

Cassileth BR. *The Alternative Medicine Handbook.* New York: W.W. Norton, 1998:122–130.

Ernst E, ed. *The Desktop Guide to Complementary and Alternative Medicine: An Evidence-Based Approach.* Edinburgh: Mosby, 2001.

Spencer JW, Jacobs JJ. *Complementary and Alternative Medicine: An Evidence-Based Approach*. St. Louis: Mosby, 2003.

Weintraub MI, Micozzi MS, eds. *Alternative and Complementary Treatments in Neurologic Illness*. New York: Churchill Livingstone, 2001, pp. 177–178.

Journal Articles

Hall H, Minnes L, Olness K. The psychophysiology of voluntary immunomodulation. *Int J Neurosci* 1993;69:221–234.

Maguire BL. The effects of imagery on attitudes and moods in multiple sclerosis patients. *Alt Ther* 1996;2:75–79.

Smith GR, McKenzie JM, Marmer DJ, et al. Psychologic modulation of the human immune response to *Varicella zoster*. *Arch Intern Med* 1985;145:221–235.

Van Fleet S. Relaxation and imagery for symptom management: improving patient assessment and individualizing treatment. *ONF* 2000;27:501–510.

23

Herbs

Herbal medicine has been used for tens of thousands of years. By about 60,000 B.C., Neanderthals apparently used two herbs, yarrow and marsh mallow, for therapeutic purposes. Within traditional Chinese medicine, herbal medicine was initially developed around 3000 B.C. and, ultimately, more than 10,000 different Chinese herbal formulas were compiled.

Herbal medicine was popular in the United States from 1820 to 1920. After 1920, herbal therapies were replaced by conventional medications. A recent resurgence of interest in herbal medicine has occurred, and herbs are currently one of the most frequently used forms of complementary and alternative medicine (CAM). The use of herbs by Americans nearly quadrupled between 1990 and 1997. In a return to earlier times, some major mainstream pharmaceutical companies are now developing and marketing herbal therapies.

Much of the popularity of herbs probably is related to the ease with which they can be used. There is no need to make an appointment with a practitioner to get started on herbal therapy. Rather, one can simply buy the herb at the local grocery store or health food store.

Herbs also have become more popular since the passage in 1994 of the Dietary Supplements Health and Education Act (DSHEA), which loosened the regulations for dietary supplements such as herbs. In fact, the regulations are so relaxed that few standards for safety, effectiveness, or quality exist. To counter some of the laxity of DSHEA, new directions for the United States market have been proposed in the *Initiative to Provide Better Health Information for Consumers*. (Information about this program is available at www.cfsan.fda.gov.) Through this program, the U.S. Food and Drug Administration (FDA) announced several objectives, including collaboration to improve the evidence base for safety and enforcement decisions, implementation of a process to evaluate safety concerns and improve the quality and consistency of products (Good Manufacturing Practices), and the mandated creation of documents with the evidence needed to make claims of effectiveness.

Herbs Contain Many Different Chemicals

An important distinction between drugs and herbs is that most drugs consist of a single chemical compound, whereas herbs consist of many different ones. Of all the chemicals in herbs, some may be beneficial, some may be harmful, and a large number have unknown effects on the human body. Fortunately, most of the chemicals are not toxic, and most are present in small enough quantities that significant harmful effects are unlikely.

Many chemicals with beneficial activity against disease have been identified in herbs. It is estimated that 25 percent of prescription drugs and 60 percent of over-the-counter drugs are derived from plants. Well-known examples of these drugs are digitalis, which is derived from the foxglove plant, and quinine, which is derived from South American Peruvian bark. Steroids, which are used to treat multiple sclerosis (MS) attacks, have a very specific chemical structure. Chemicals with steroid-like structures and biologic effects have been identified in Asian ginseng (ginsenoside) and in licorice (glycyrrhizic acid).

Herbs may contain chemicals that have harmful effects. For example, the lily-of-the-valley plant contains potent heart toxins. Some herbs, such as chaparral and comfrey (or contaminants mixed in with the herbs), have been associated with a severe liver toxicity that has led to death or the need for liver transplantation. An example of a tragic case of liver injury was described in February 1999. A 28-year-old man with mild MS was treating his disease with zinc and two herbal medicines, scullcap and pau d'arco. He developed severe liver injury and died. The liver injury was believed to be due to a chemical contaminant in the scullcap.

Fortunately, most of the chemicals in herbs do not have toxic effects. For most herbs, the majority of the chemicals probably have neither beneficial nor harmful properties; if demonstrated beneficial effects of an herb exist, they probably are due to one or several of the many chemicals present. Thus, for many herbs, it is likely that one or a few chemicals could be producing a beneficial effect and that the remaining chemicals do not have any beneficial or harmful effects.

It is sometimes claimed that herbs cannot have harmful effects because the chemicals in them are present in such small quantities. It is also claimed that herbs have beneficial qualities. These two statements are not consistent with each other. *If a therapy is strong enough to produce beneficial effects, it usually is also strong enough to produce harmful effects.* As more research is conducted, it may indeed be found that, relative to prescription medications, herbs generally have fewer side effects, but are also somewhat less effective.

Important Features of Herbs

Most herbs have not been studied as extensively as have drugs. As a result, it is often not known exactly which chemicals in herbs are the active ingredients. Similarly, the side effects of herbs and their interactions with drugs are not fully understood. In summary, even for well-studied herbs, the full range of effectiveness and the full range of side effects are not completely known.

Another important aspect of herbs is their variability. Because of the current lack of strict regulation in the United States, a great deal of variability is present in the quantity of the presumed active ingredient present in different herbal preparations. For example, one study of ginseng found 50 times as much of the active ingredient in some products as in others; this situation is similar to a physician telling a patient to take somewhere between one and 50 pills for a medical condition! Other reports have found no active ingredient in some ginseng preparations.

Finally, herbs should be avoided in certain circumstances. People should avoid herbs if they have multiple medical problems or are taking multiple medications; women who are pregnant or breast-feeding and children also should avoid herbs. Some medications have a very specific range in which they are effective and in which they do not have side effects. These include anticonvulsant medications, blood-thinning medications, and some heart medications. Herbs should not be taken with these medications because we do not know all of possible interactions that herbs could have with them. Some herbs could mildly alter the blood levels of these medications and thereby decrease their effectiveness or increase their side effects.

Herbal Therapy Guidelines

The most conservative approach to the use of herbs in MS is to state that they should be avoided entirely. The basis for this argument is that the effects of herbs have not been directly studied in MS, and it is therefore possible that an herb now thought to be safe could through future research be found to adversely affect the MS disease process.

For those interested in considering herb use, guidelines can make decision-making easier. These guidelines are outlined in Table 23.1. The final principle is very important—always discuss the use of herbs with your physician.

TABLE 23.1. *Herbal Therapy Guidelines*

- Herbs are often used as drugs.
- Herbs contain many different compounds, some of which may be toxic or interact with drugs.
- Herbs may contain compounds that have not yet been identified or characterized.
- The quality and composition of herbal preparations are variable.
- Herbs generally should be used for a short time for benign, self-limited conditions.
- Herbs should be avoided in women who are pregnant or breast-feeding.
- Herbs should be avoided by people who have multiple medical problems or are taking multiple medications.
- Use caution and discuss herbal use with a physician before starting.

Choose Reliable Herb Suppliers

When using herbs, it is important to purchase them from companies that produce high-quality, consistent preparations. Some of the highest quality preparations are produced in Europe. Brands chosen should be standardized and contain specified amounts of active ingredients. The product also should list other specific information: common and scientific name of the herb, the manufacturer's name and address, batch and lot number, expiration date, dose recommendations, potential side effects, and quality control information. Higher-quality herbal products in the United States have the symbols for the United States Pharmacopeia (USP) or the National Formulary (NF). To evaluate the quality of some herbs and other dietary supplement products, independent laboratory evaluations of products have been done by *Consumer Reports* and by an organization known as *Consumerlab.com* (www.consumerlab.com). The results of these evaluations are available from these sources.

Consideration of Specific Herbs

Many different herbal preparations are available. To provide practical information in this area, this section reviews some of the most popular herbs in the United States. Herbs with particular relevance to MS also are reviewed. These herbs are presented in alphabetical order. Following this section, both common and uncommon herbs are discussed in terms of their possible effects on MS and possible interactions with medications frequently used to manage MS.

Herbs Commonly Used in the General Population and Herbs That Are Relevant to MS

Coffee and Other Caffeine-Containing Herbs and Supplements

Coffee, perhaps not generally thought of as an herb, is in fact one of the most popular herbs in the world. Its effects on mental alertness and fatigue are well known to those who drink their regular morning cup of coffee. The effects of coffee are due to one of its chemical constituents, caffeine. In addition to coffee, other herbs and supplements contain caffeine.

Coffee is of interest for people with MS because of its possible effects on fatigue. No systematic approaches exist to using coffee or other caffeine-containing herbs in people with MS. Despite the fairly widespread use of caffeine products by people with MS, very little research has been done in this area.

The largest study to date was conducted by the Rocky Mountain Multiple Sclerosis Center—the results of this study have been published in a preliminary form (1) and may be viewed at www.ms.cam.org, the CAM website of the Rocky Mountain MS Center. This study was an online survey that involved nearly 2,000 people with MS. Those who appeared to have MS fatigue were questioned about the various conventional and unconventional therapies that they had tried. For the respondents, about 50 percent believed that some form of caffeine was helpful for their fatigue. Another MS study that included caffeine involved a therapy known as *Prokarin*—the results of this study are difficult to interpret for several reasons, including the fact that Prokarin contains caffeine as well as histamine (see the chapter on Prokarin).

In the general population, strong evidence suggests that coffee improves mental alertness, thereby potentially improving mental fatigue. In contrast, coffee does not appear to improve physical power or endurance and therefore probably does not have a beneficial effect on physical fatigue.

Another area of possible relevance to MS is immune system alteration by caffeine. Some studies indicate that caffeine may decrease the activity of lymphocytes, a type of immune system cell, and produce changes in a protein in the brain known as the *adenosine receptor*. In theory, these effects could be beneficial for MS, but studies in this area are too preliminary to allow any definite conclusions.

Other herbal sources of caffeine exist. Tea contains a significant amount of caffeine. In the United States, black tea, derived from the leaves of *Camellia sinensis*, is the most popular form. Green tea is prepared from the same plant, but the leaves are processed differently. Another well-known source of caffeine is chocolate and other food products derived from the cacao plant. Cola nut, also known as kola nut and bissy nut, contains caffeine. Guarana is a South American caffeine-containing herb that may be consumed as a tea or in tablet form. Another South American herb that contains caffeine, maté or yerba maté, is not especially popular in the United States but is popular in some South American countries. Finally, the most direct approach is to take caffeine itself, which is available in tablet form as a dietary supplement.

The amount of caffeine available from these products is variable. A convenient reference point to start with is a 6-ounce cup of percolated coffee, which contains approximately 100 milligrams of caffeine. It is important to note that less caffeine is present in instant coffee and darker roast coffees, including latté, cappuccino, and other popular espresso-based coffees. In comparison to a typical cup of coffee, approximately one-half the amount of caffeine (30 to 60 milligrams) may be obtained from a cup of tea, cocoa, or maté; a 12-ounce bottle of a cola drink; or an 800-milligram tablet of guarana. Relatively low amounts of caffeine (5 to 10 mg) typically are contained in a chocolate bar. Caffeine tablets often contain 100 or 200 milligrams of caffeine and are roughly equivalent to one or two cups of coffee.

The frequency with which one ingests caffeine may influence the herb's ability to improve mental alertness. With high levels of fatigue in the morning, people often drink extra cups of coffee at that time. However, research indicates that this may not be the most effective approach. It has been reported that small amounts of caffeine (about 20 milligrams or about one-fifth of a cup of coffee) taken on an hourly basis may be especially effective for promoting wakefulness.

The FDA regards coffee and other caffeine-containing herbs as generally safe. One precaution to be aware of is the possible effect of caffeine on a developing fetus. Because of this concern, the FDA recommends that pregnant women avoid or limit caffeine consumption. Maté is an herb that has raised concern. Studies indicate that maté, especially in high doses, may increase the risk of cancers of the mouth, throat, kidney, bladder, and lung. Notably, two North American forms of maté, *Ilex cassine* and *Ilex vomitoria*, are classified as not safe by the FDA.

Some specific concerns exist about MS and caffeine-containing products. Caffeine use may worsen MS-associated bladder problems because it increases urination and may irritate the urinary tract. Caffeine use may increase the risk of osteoporosis, a condition to which people with MS may be especially prone. In addition, theoretical risks are associated with the use of high doses of green tea. This form of tea contains relatively high levels of antioxidants, which, in theory, may stimulate the immune system (see "Vitamins, Minerals, and Other Nonherbal Supplements"); this effect may be harmful for people with MS.

High doses of caffeine should be avoided because they may produce anxiety, insomnia, heart palpitations, upset stomach, nausea, vomiting, high blood pressure, tremors, muscle twitching, and increased cholesterol levels. The long-term use of large doses of caffeine may lead to an addiction-type situation in which higher and higher doses are required for the same effect and in which abrupt discontinuation causes mild withdrawal symptoms such as headache, irritability, dizziness, and anxiety. The safety of caffeine in women who are pregnant or breast-feeding is unclear.

Caffeine-containing preparations also interact with other supplements and medications. Simultaneously taking moderate doses of two or three caffeine-containing supplements may lead to excessive levels of caffeine. Also, both the stimulant actions and the adverse effects of caffeine may be accentuated when it is consumed with *ma huang* (ephedra) or with grapefruit juice. The blood levels of caffeine may be increased by multiple medications, including oral contraceptives, cimetidine (Tagamet), and verapamil (Calan).

The usual maximum daily dose of caffeine is 250 to 300 milligrams. This is equivalent to two to three cups of coffee or four to five cups of tea. The timing and dose of caffeine that may be most beneficial for MS-related fatigue has not been studied.

Cranberry and Other Herbal Therapies for Urinary Tract Infections

Cranberry juice is of relevance because urinary tract infections (UTIs) are common with MS, and cranberry juice has a long history of use in their prevention and treatment. From the 1920s to the 1970s, it was believed that the acid from cranberry juice makes the urine acidic and that this increase in acidity prevents and treats UTIs. However, subsequent studies showed that the effect of cranberry juice was probably due to the presence of two types of compounds, fructose and a class of chemicals known as proanthocyanidins. These chemicals do not destroy bacteria. Instead, they appear to keep bacteria from attaching to the walls of the urinary tract. As a result, it is believed that bacteria present in the urinary tract are unable to cause an infection and are simply passed in the urine. In addition to these effects, cranberry juice, like antibiotic medications, also may kill some bacteria.

Limited clinical studies indicate that cranberry may prevent UTIs in some people. A beneficial effect has been reported in studies of UTI prevention in women who have normal bladder function. However, limited studies of people with abnormal bladder function, which may occur in MS, indicate that cranberry is *not* effective for UTI prevention. A rigorous, well-designed study of cranberry use for the prevention or treatment of UTIs has not been done yet. Also, it is not known how the effectiveness of cranberry compares with that of prescription antibiotics, the more conventional method for preventing UTIs.

Because UTIs in people with MS may lead to serious complications, including worsening of neurologic difficulties, cranberry juice should not be used to treat infections. On the other hand, for people interested in an herbal approach, it may be reasonable to attempt to *prevent* infections using cranberry juice. The exact doses that should be used have not been established. Doses sometimes recommended for prevention are 1 to 10 ounces of juice daily. Six capsules of dried powder or 1.5 ounces of frozen or fresh cranberries may be equivalent to 3 ounces of juice. The use of frozen or fresh cranberries may not be possible because of the sour taste of the berries. Cranberry juice cocktail is 26 to 33 percent juice.

Cranberry generally is well tolerated. Cranberry may interact with blood-thinning medications, including warfarin (Coumadin). The chronic use of high doses may increase the risk of developing kidney stones and may cause stomach discomfort, loose stools, and nausea. The safety of cranberry use in women who are pregnant or breast-feeding is not known.

Another herb sometimes recommended for UTIs is bearberry, also known as uva ursi. Some concerns about this herb exist. Specifically, it is not clearly effective for UTI prevention, it appears to be less effective with acidic urine, it may cause nausea and vomiting, and it contains chemicals that may have cancer-causing properties.

Taking vitamin C supplements is a nonherbal approach sometimes recommended for preventing and treating UTIs. However, clinical studies do not support the use of vitamin C for preventing or treating these infections. Vitamin C may increase the risk of kidney stones in those with a history of kidney stones. A theoretical risk exists that high doses of vitamin C may stimulate the immune system and possibly worsen MS.

Echinacea

Echinacea is one of the most popular and well-studied herbs. A long history of echinacea use exists for the treatment of medical conditions, especially infections. North American Indians used echinacea medicinally, and it was the primary herbal therapy for infections in the early 1900s. Echinacea poses a theoretical risk for people with MS, yet, surprisingly, it is sometimes recommended for MS and appears to be used by a relatively large number of people with the disease.

Echinacea is of interest to people with MS because it may prevent or reduce the severity of viral infections. Because viral infections may, in some instances, provoke an MS attack, their reduction has obvious potential benefit. Also, popular books on alternative medicine sometimes specifically recommend echinacea as a treatment for MS, possibly because of echinacea's effects on the immune system.

Many scientific and clinical studies have evaluated echinacea. Some, but not all, studies indicate that echinacea limits the duration and severity of infections, especially the common cold.

The important point for people with MS is that echinacea may act by stimulating two components of the immune system, *macrophages* and *T cells*. Macrophages and T cells are already excessively active in MS, and MS medications, such as glatiramer acetate (Copaxone) and interferons (Avonex, Betaseron, and Rebif), decrease their activity. Thus, consuming echinacea may conceivably worsen MS by further stimulating these immune cells, and this may decrease the effectiveness of MS medications. One report documents a person who developed an MS-like condition known as *acute disseminated encephalomyelitis* (ADEM) after being treated with an herbal muscle injection that included echinacea. Theoretical concerns exist that echinacea may produce liver injury. This effect could be increased if echinacea is taken with those MS medications having possible toxic effects on the liver, including interferons (Avonex, Betaseron, and Rebif) and methotrexate, a chemotherapy drug sometimes used to treat MS. *In summary, it is safest for people with MS to avoid echinacea.*

What about other measures to prevent or treat the common cold or other minor infections? Goldenseal and garlic (see subsequent sections) have not been shown to have definite effects on infections, and the scientific basis for their use is unclear. Also, vitamin C and zinc, which are discussed in detail elsewhere in this book, sometimes are used for infections. However, both of these compounds also have unclear effects on infections and may activate the immune system.

People with MS may take several safe measures to prevent and treat viral infections such as the flu and common cold. First, the flu vaccine is readily available, appears to be safe for people with MS, and helps prevent the flu. Recently developed prescription medications (oseltamivir [Tamiflu], zanamivir [Relenza]) also decrease the severity of the flu. Finally, viral infections may be prevented by simple measures such as avoiding contact with people with viral infections and frequent hand-washing.

Evening Primrose Oil

See the chapter "Diets and Fatty Acid Supplements."

Garlic

Over the past 25 years, more than 1,000 studies have evaluated the possible therapeutic effects of garlic. Suggestive, but not conclusive, results have been obtained in studies of the effectiveness of garlic in treating high cholesterol levels, high blood pressure, and cancer. On the basis of limited scientific studies, garlic sometimes is recommended as a treatment for the common cold.

With regard to MS, some research has shown that garlic may stimulate two types of immune cells, macrophages and lymphocytes. No clinical studies have directly evaluated the effect of garlic on MS or other autoimmune diseases. However, on a theoretical basis, garlic could adversely affect the course of MS through its immune-stimulating activity.

Controversy exists regarding the best form and dose of garlic. Some commercial preparations actually contain none of the presumed active chemical, *allicin*. Garlic may inhibit blood clotting and thus should be avoided in people with blood-clotting disorders, people undergoing surgery, and people taking blood-thinning medications or aspirin.

Ginkgo biloba

Ginkgo biloba has been evaluated in many human clinical studies and has the honor of being the most extensively studied herb. *Ginkgo biloba* usually refers to the extract derived from the leaf of the *Ginkgo biloba* tree. This herb is sometimes recommended as a therapy for MS.

Some of the more recent popularity of *Ginkgo biloba* may be due to an investigation published in 1997 in the *Journal of the American Medical Association* (*JAMA*). In this study, *Ginkgo biloba* extract was found to be effective in treating cognitive difficulties in the elderly.

Several biological effects have been associated with *Ginkgo biloba*. Some of its chemical constituents act as antioxidants, while others inhibit the effects of platelet-activating factor (PAF), a compound in the body that plays a role in inflammation and blood clotting.

Because of the inflammatory effect of PAF, it and *Ginkgo biloba* have been studied in MS. In animals with EAE, an experimental model of MS, PAF worsens the disease, whereas *Ginkgo biloba*, in some but not all studies, produces improvement. On the basis of these findings in animals, a small study, reported in 1992, examined the effects of *Ginkgo biloba* on MS attacks and found that eight of ten people improved using *Ginkgo biloba* treatment. Some herbal medicine and CAM books recommend *Ginkgo biloba* for MS because of the results of this study. It is sometimes not mentioned that this encouraging 1992 study was, unfortunately, followed by a 1995 study that found *Ginkgo biloba* ineffective for treating MS attacks.

The 1995 study, which involved 104 people, was better designed and involved a larger number of patients than did the 1992 study. *Thus*, Ginkgo biloba *does not appear to be effective for the short-term treatment of MS attacks.* It is not known whether *Ginkgo biloba* decreases MS disease activity when it is used on a long-term, as opposed to short-term, basis.

Two preliminary studies have been done on the effects of *Ginkgo biloba* on cognition in people with MS. Both these studies produced positive results. Further research is needed to clarify whether *Ginkgo biloba* has definite therapeutic effects on MS-related cognitive difficulties.

Ginkgo biloba usually is well tolerated. If this herb is used, it is important to keep in mind that it has a tendency to increase bleeding. Spontaneous bleeding around the brain or in the eye has been described in a few patients taking this herb. It probably should be avoided by people who take blood-thinning medications (warfarin or Coumadin) or aspirin, people who have bleeding disorders, and people who are undergoing surgery. *Ginkgo biloba* may increase the risk of seizures and thus should be used with caution by those with seizures. *Ginkgo biloba* may also cause rashes, dizziness, headache, and gastrointestinal symptoms, including nausea, vomiting, diarrhea, and flatulence. It is not known if ginkgo is safe in women who are pregnant or breast-feeding.

Clinical studies of *Ginkgo biloba* generally use standardized leaf extracts. In these preparations, known in Germany as EGb 761 and LI 1370, a specific content of certain chemicals (24 to 25 percent flavone glycosides and 6 percent terpene lactones) is present. Commercially available products referred to as EGb 761 include Tebonin, Tanakan, and Rokan. Products referred to as LI 1371 include Kaveri, Kaver, Ginkgold (Nature's Way), Ginkoba (Pharmaton), and Quanterra Mental Sharpness.

Ginseng

Several different types of ginseng are available. Asian ginseng (*Panax ginseng*), is the most common and most extensively studied form. Another type of ginseng is Siberian ginseng or eleuthero (*Eleutherococcus senticosus*).

Both Asian ginseng and Siberian ginseng are derived from roots. They are referred to as *adaptogens*, which means that they are believed to increase resistance to stress and increase energy levels. Although the effects of these herbs may be desired by many people with MS, it is not clear that consuming either of them is the best way to produce these effects.

Asian ginseng has been associated with many different biological actions. *Ginsenosides*, which may be the active constituents in Asian ginseng, have a chemical structure similar to that of steroids, which are used to treat MS attacks and *suppress* the immune system. Paradoxically, *activation* of the immune system also has been associated with Asian ginseng. Multiple studies have shown that the herb stimulates immune system cells, including T cells and macrophages. On the basis of these immune-system effects, Asian ginseng has been investigated as a possible treatment for cancer and AIDS. Clinical studies of the effects of Asian ginseng on stress and fatigue have yielded mixed results.

Although Siberian ginseng is an entirely different herb from Asian ginseng, research on Siberian ginseng has produced results similar to that on Asian ginseng. Specifically, scientific research on the herb indicates that it may have immune-stimulating properties, and clinical studies do not definitely show beneficial effects on stress and fatigue.

Side effects and drug interactions are possible with the use of Asian ginseng and Siberian ginseng. Both herbs may produce sedation and may conceivably worsen MS fatigue or accentuate the sedating effects of medications and alcohol. Asian ginseng may interact with steroids, which sometimes are used to treat MS attacks. Asian ginseng and Siberian ginseng may increase bleeding tendency and should be avoided by people who are undergoing surgery, people who have blood-clotting disorders, and people who take blood-thinning medications or aspirin.

Because Asian ginseng and Siberian ginseng may activate the immune system and have not been shown to have definite clinical benefits, it is reasonable for people with MS to avoid high doses and the regular use of these herbs.

Goldenseal

Goldenseal has been used medicinally for at least 200 years. This herb is taken alone or in combination with echinacea for a variety of infections, including the common cold. Unlike echinacea, which has been investigated extensively, little recent information is available about the biological effects or possible clinical benefits of goldenseal or its chemical constituents, berberine and hydrastine. Because of the limited information about goldenseal, it is difficult to make any definite conclusions about this herb. The clinical studies to date do not support its use for infections. Notably, goldenseal may produce sedation. Therefore, it may worsen MS fatigue or increase the sedating effects of alcohol and some prescription medications.

Grape Seed Extract

Grape seed extract use has grown in popularity recently. It is sold for its antioxidant activity; grape seed extract contains complex mixtures of chemicals known as *oligomeric proanthocyanidins* or *OPCs*. These chemicals are similar to those in pycnogenol and act as antioxidants. Some studies indicate that the chemicals in grape seed extract are more potent antioxidants than are vitamin C or vitamin E.

The clinical use of grape seed extract has not been studied extensively. A preliminary report indicates that grape seed extract treatment of the animal model of MS decreases the severity of the disease on the basis of several measures. Grape seed extract also decreased the number of immune cells entering the central nervous system, inhibited an enzyme that allows immune cells to enter the central nervous system, and decreased levels of inflammation-related immune molecules. These results are encouraging and may lead to human studies of grape seed extract in MS.

Based on current information, for people with MS who want to take antioxidants, it may be best to take low doses of inexpensive antioxidant vitamins, such as vitamin A (beta-carotene), vitamin C, and vitamin E (see the chapter on "Vitamins, Minerals, and Nonherbal Supplements").

Kava Kava

Kava kava is an herb that has been used in the Pacific islands for hundreds of years for its purported relaxant effects. It is one of the few herbs for which the active chemicals have been identified. These chemicals, known as *kavalactones* or *kavapyrones*, interact with proteins in the central nervous system that are known as *GABA-A receptors*. These are the same proteins that mediate the effects of diazepam (Valium) and related anti-anxiety drugs. Several studies indicate that kava kava decreases mild anxiety. It does not appear to be effective for more severe forms of anxiety.

Kava kava sometimes is recommended for insomnia. However, its effects on insomnia have not been well studied. Another herb, valerian, has been more extensively studied for insomnia than kava kava (see the section on Valerian).

Most drugs that decrease anxiety also produce sedation. Surprisingly, kava kava itself does not appear to have this effect. However, kava kava may increase the sedating effects of alcohol and several medications that are frequently used in MS, including lioresal (Baclofen), tizanidine (Zanaflex), and diazepam (Valium). The effects of kava kava on MS fatigue are not known. Heavy use of kava kava over months may produce skin problems, red eyes, itching, and other difficulties.

Until recently, kava kava was thought to be generally well tolerated. In 2001, however, several reports surfaced of liver toxicity in association with kava kava use. Subsequently, more than 50 reports appeared of kava kava–associated liver toxicity. In some cases, people died or required liver transplants. Kava kava is now banned in Europe and Canada. In the United

States, the FDA has issued warnings about the herb. Due to these safety issues, kava kava should not be used.

Padma 28

Padma 28, also known as Badmaev 28 and Gabyr-Nirynga, is a complex mixture of herbs sometimes recommended for MS. This herbal combination was developed in the late nineteenth century in the Buryat region of the Russian Empire by two physicians, Sul-Tim-Badma and Zham-Saram-Badma, also known as Dr. Alexander Badmaev and Dr. Peter Badmaev. The practices of these physicians were influenced by traditions of Ayurvedic and Tibetan medicine. Padma 28 is taken by mouth and contains more than 20 different herbs and calcium. It appears to have antioxidant effects and may mildly decrease immune system activity.

Padma 28 has been claimed to be effective for MS and other conditions, including heart disease, peripheral vascular disease, and asthma. In mice with EAE, an animal form of MS, consuming water that contains Padma 28 is associated with longer survival times and decreased death rates. A 1992 study in Poland evaluated Padma 28 treatment in 100 people with a progressive form of MS (2). Over the course of a year, one group of people received Padma 28 and the other group received no herbal treatment. In the treated group, 44 percent had some type of clinical improvement; none of the untreated people improved. This study is promising, but because specific details of its design are not available, the strength of the effect is not entirely clear.

The 1992 Polish study of 100 people reported no side effects. No other detailed toxicity information about Padma 28 is available.

Limited studies with Padma 28 suggest that it may be beneficial for MS. However, these studies are by no means conclusive, and limited information is available on the safety of this herbal preparation, especially for long-term use.

Psyllium, Bran, and Other Herbs for Constipation

Psyllium is an herb used to relieve constipation. It is of potential importance to people with MS because constipation is a relatively frequent symptom of the disease.

Clinical studies have shown that psyllium effectively treats constipation. Unlike most other herbs, psyllium is approved by the FDA. It is referred to as a "bulk-producing laxative" because it increases in size, or bulk, when it comes in contact with water. Psyllium, probably the most popular bulk-producing laxative, is used daily in some form by approximately four million Americans.

Psyllium is a form of dietary fiber. Recent studies with psyllium and other sources of fiber have shown that a high fiber intake may improve several medical conditions, including high cholesterol levels, heart disease, and hypertension.

Psyllium usually is well tolerated. However, the FDA warns that it may produce choking, especially if the intake of fluids is not adequate or an individual has swallowing difficulties. Notably, some people with MS *do* have swallowing difficulties, and they should avoid using psyllium seed or husk.

Psyllium is available in over-the-counter preparations such as Metamucil. It also may be taken in the form of the seed or husk. The FDA recommends that each dose of psyllium be taken with at least 8 ounces of water or other fluid. Oral medications should be taken 1 hour before or 4 hours after psyllium, because psyllium may alter the absorption of these drugs.

Other herbal therapies are available for constipation. One source of fiber is bran, the outer coat of grains, including wheat, oats, and rice. Bran may be consumed as a breakfast cereal, in tablet form, or as crude fiber. Other fiber-rich foods include apples, citrus fruits, and beans. Other herbs that appear to be effective for relieving constipation and are generally safe for short-term use (1 to 2 weeks) include buckthorn, cascara, castor oil, guar gum, olive oil, and senna. The long-term use of some of these herbs may lead to dependence on their use and decreased blood levels of potassium.

Pycnogenol

Pycnogenol has been used as a dietary supplement for approximately 15 years. It is made from the bark of the French maritime pine tree. Pycnogenol is a mixture of chemicals known as *oligomeric proanthocyanidins* (OPCs). These chemicals, which are similar to those in grape seed extract and green tea leaves, appear to act as antioxidants.

Pycnogenol has been touted as a treatment for many diseases, including MS. At this time, however, no formal clinical studies have evaluated its effects on MS. A preliminary report indicates that grape seed extract, which contains OPCs, decreases disease severity in the animal model of MS. Further research on the effects on MS of pycnogenol, OPCs, and antioxidants generally is needed.

Pycnogenol may have several immune-system effects, which may be the result of its antioxidant activity. As with other antioxidant supplements, it is not clear whether increased antioxidant activity is necessarily beneficial for MS (see the chapter "Vitamins, Minerals, and Other Nonherbal

Supplements"). The safety of long-term pycnogenol use has not been documented in the general population. Pycnogenol and other specialized antioxidant preparations generally are more expensive than are antioxidant vitamins.

Based on current evidence, no compelling reason exists for people with MS to use pycnogenol. If antioxidant supplements are taken by people with MS, it may be most logical (and most economical) to take low doses of one or more antioxidant vitamins, such as vitamin A (or beta-carotene), vitamin C, and vitamin E.

St. John's Wort

St. John's wort has been used for therapeutic purposes for more than 2,000 years. Its most common current use is as an antidepressant.

Although St. John's wort has been studied extensively, the chemicals that may produce its effects have not been clearly identified. In the past, it was thought that a chemical known as hypericin may be responsible for its effects. However, more recent studies indicate that another chemical, hyperforin, may play an important role. In addition to uncertainties about its active constituents, it is not known how this herb alters brain function. Hyperforin affects multiple chemicals in the brain, including serotonin, norepinephrine, and dopamine. Effects on hormones and even the immune system have been proposed. In the end, St. John's wort (and other herbs) may be found to exert multiple biologic effects.

Many studies have investigated the antidepressant effects of St. John's wort. One study was a combined analysis of 27 different studies that included a total of 2,291 patients. This study indicates that St. John's wort produces antidepressant effects in people with mild to moderate depression. The quality of some of these clinical studies has been criticized. Of note, it is not clear if St. John's wort is effective for those with severe depression.

To clarify the possible role of St. John's wort as an antidepressant, two recent studies were conducted. Although the results were negative, there were limitations to these studies. Specifically, one of the studies evaluated the effects of placebo, St. John's wort, and sertraline (Zoloft). St. John's wort was no more effective than placebo, but the same was true for Zoloft. Also, this study evaluated people with severe depression, as opposed to mild to moderate depression. In the other study, placebo and St. John's wort were compared in people with mild to moderate depression. Once again, St. John's wort produced results similar to those of placebo—this study may not have had enough "power" to detect a difference between the placebo and St. John's wort groups.

Because of the association of MS with depression, St. John's wort may be considered for use by people with MS. No studies have directly evaluated its use in MS. Interestingly, some studies indicate that St. John's wort decreases the levels of interleukin-6 (IL-6), an immune-system chemical that activates the immune system and may be involved in the flulike side effects of the interferons (Avonex, Betaseron, and Rebif).

Several factors should be kept in mind when considering treatment with St. John's wort. First, depression should be discussed with a physician, because it is not a condition that people should diagnose and treat on their own. St. John's wort should not be used for severe depression (as opposed to mild or moderate depression). Although this herb is generally well tolerated, it may occasionally produce side effects, including upset stomach, sedation, dizziness, irritability, anxiety, and confusion. Rarely, St. John's wort may produce sensitivity of the skin and nerves to sun exposure (photosensitivity), especially in fair-skinned people. In those with depression or manic-depressive illness, St. John's wort may provoke conditions known as *mania* and *hypomania*, which are characterized by excessive physical and mental activity. Abrupt discontinuation of St. John's wort may cause withdrawal side effects, including headache, nausea, dizziness, insomnia, confusion, and fatigue.

Important potential drug interactions occur with St. John's wort. Because of its effects on the liver, St. John's wort may decrease the blood levels of a variety of prescription medications. These medications include oral contraceptives. (This has led some to say that some "little St. Johns" may be running around now because of unexpected pregnancies that occurred with the combined use of oral contraceptives and St. John's wort.) Other drugs that may be affected by St. John's wort include medications commonly used to treat heart disease, depression, seizures, and cancer. Among these drugs of concern, several are used for MS-related symptoms: alprazolam (Xanax), carbamazepine (Tegretol), imipramine (Tofranil), phenytoin (Dilantin), phenobarbital, and primidone (Mysoline). St. John's wort may decrease blood levels of blood-thinning medication (warfarin or Coumadin). In addition, the herb should not be taken in conjunction with antidepressant medications, including those referred to as tricyclic antidepressants (such as nortriptyline [Pamelor] and amitriptyline [Elavil]), selective serotonin reuptake inhibitors (SSRIs) such as fluoxetine (Prozac), paroxetine (Paxil), and sertraline (Zoloft), and monoamine oxidase (MAO) inhibitors.

Tablets of St. John's wort are usually 300 milligrams. Tablets should be standardized to contain 0.3 percent hypericin. In most studies, 300 milligrams has been given three times daily.

Spirulina

People have consumed Spirulina, also known as blue-green algae, for hundreds of years. It was harvested from lakes near Mexico City by the Aztecs and from Lake Chad by natives of the Sahara Desert.

Spirulina sometimes is recommended for MS. It also is claimed to be effective for many other conditions, including fatigue, cancer, obesity, arthritis, viral infections, high cholesterol levels, and hair loss. Spirulina is also known as "super seaweed" and "superfood." It is rich in vitamins, minerals, and proteins, and is available in tablets, capsules, powders, and processed foods such as snack bars. It produces a characteristic intense green color when added to drinks.

It is not entirely clear why Spirulina is recommended for MS. Vitamin B_{12} supplements are sometimes suggested for people with MS, and Spirulina contains a form of vitamin B_{12}. However, it is not clear whether vitamin B_{12} is beneficial for most people with MS. Also, it appears that much of the vitamin B_{12} in Spirulina is in a chemical form not utilized by the human body and may antagonize the effects of active forms of vitamin B_{12}.

One particular species of Spirulina contains gamma-linolenic acid (GLA), which could possibly be beneficial for MS (see the chapter on "Diets and Fatty Acid Supplements"), but many other species of Spirulina do not contain GLA, and it is hard to know which species are present in any given Spirulina product.

Spirulina may be associated with MS therapy because some studies have determined that it acts on the immune system. However, these immune-system effects have been variable and of unclear significance. Some studies indicate that Spirulina stimulates the immune system and thus, theoretically, may actually be harmful for MS. Isolated reports suggest that in individuals with other immune conditions (pemphigus vulgaris, dermatomyositis), symptoms may be provoked by Spirulina. Finally, Spirulina may be recommended for MS because it is claimed to be effective for fatigue. No well-documented published studies support this claim.

In addition to the lack of evidence supporting its use specifically in MS, Spirulina is relatively expensive, and its safety is not known. Spirulina is at least 10 to 20 times more costly than other protein sources, such as beef and milk. Insufficient information is available about the safety of long-term Spirulina use. Although it has been consumed in some countries for hundreds of years with no apparent adverse effects, some batches of Spirulina have been found to contain mercury, lead, arsenic, radioactive metals, bird feathers, flies, and microbes. Contaminated products may cause nausea, vomiting, liver toxicity, and death.

Stinging Nettle

The stinging nettle plant has been used traditionally in folk medicine. It is currently sometimes recommended for MS, urinary tract infections, and many other medical conditions. Nettle is notable for having stinging hairs containing chemicals that produce skin irritation.

Nettle may have some therapeutic effects. For example, it may have anti-inflammmatory and pain-relieving actions. However, no clinical studies justify the use of nettle for MS. In addition, scientific studies indicate that nettle may activate the immune system cells known as T cells. These effects pose theoretical risks for people with MS.

The safety of nettle has not been extensively studied. In the United States, it is classified as an herb of "undefined safety." Nettle may produce sedation, and thus has the potential to worsen MS fatigue and increase the effects of sedating medications and alcohol. Because of its vitamin K content, nettle may interfere with the effects of blood-thinning medications such as warfarin or Coumadin.

Valerian

Valerian has been used as a sedating and calming herb for over 1,000 years. It is sometimes referred to as "the Valium of the nineteenth century." Valerian has a characteristic odor, which is similar to that of dirty socks. A "stink rating" is sometimes used to evaluate different valerian products.

Valerian may produce its effects by an action similar to that of Valium (diazepam) and related prescription drugs (benzodiazepines). However, the active chemicals and their exact biological activities have not been determined. Ten clinical studies over the past 20 years have suggested that valerian is effective for insomnia. These studies are of variable quality.

Valerian sometimes is suggested as a treatment for anxiety, depression, and muscle stiffness (spasticity). However, due to limited clinical studies, its effects on these conditions are not known. For anxiety, more extensive studies have been done using kava kava (see preceding section) than valerian.

Sleep disorders are common in MS and may contribute to MS-associated fatigue. Sleeping difficulties may be associated with stress and anxiety. Because of the complexities of diagnosing and treating sleep disorders, this condition should be discussed with a physician.

Although valerian usually is well tolerated, the safety of long-term use has not been established. Valerian may produce excessive sedation or worsen MS fatigue, especially if it is used in combination with other sedating medications (such as lioresal [Baclofen], tizanidine [Zanaflex], and diazepam [Valium]) or alcohol. Other side effects include headache, excitability, insomnia, and possible liver toxicity.

Variable doses are given for valerian products. A typical recommended dose is 400 to 900 milligrams of valerian extract 60 to 90 minutes before bedtime. Valerian also may be taken as a tea (1 teaspoon of crude dried herb several times daily) or tincture (0.5 to 1 teaspoon) several times daily. The therapeutic effects of valerian may require daily use for 2 to 4 weeks (as opposed to sporadic use on an "as needed" basis).

Yohimbe and Yohimbine

Yohimbe refers to the bark obtained from a West African evergreen tree, which traditionally has been used for sexual disorders and as an aphrodisiac. Yohimbine is one the major chemicals present in yohimbe.

Limited studies have evaluated the effectiveness and safety of yohimbe for sexual disorders. Some studies indicate that yohimbe may be beneficial for erectile dysfunction in men and decreased libido in women. However, it has many serious side effects, including severely decreased blood pressure, abnormalities of heart rhythm (arrhythmias), heart failure, and death. Other side effects include insomnia, anxiety, tremor, high blood pressure, rapid heart rate, headache, nausea, and vomiting. The FDA has determined that yohimbe is not safe or effective and that it should not be available for over-the-counter use. Yohimbine, the active ingredient in yohimbe, is available by prescription in the United States.

People with MS may experience sexual disorders, including difficulties with erections and decreased libido. These sexual problems should be evaluated and treated by a physician or other health care professional. Yohimbine should only be used with physician supervision. For erectile dysfunction, conventional medical medications are safer and more effective than yohimbe or yohimbine.

Herbs That May Affect MS, Interact with Medications Used in MS, or Have Serious Side Effects

Many different herbs are available in the United States, especially in stores that specialize in herbal products. Their beneficial effects are sometimes described extensively, although the possible harmful effects on a specific disease such as MS are not mentioned. In this section, we consider herbs that may stimulate the immune system, worsen MS-associated symptoms, and interact with medications commonly used for MS. Potentially dangerous herbs also are discussed.

Immune-Stimulating Herbs

In scientific studies, many herbs have been shown to potentially activate the immune system (Table 23.2). Some of these herbs may stimulate immune system function through the action of a type of sugar molecule known as a polysaccharide.

The immune system has two components: the *cellular* immune system and the *humoral* immune system. The immune-stimulating effects of herbs may occur on one or both of these components. Although much MS research focuses on abnormalities in the cellular system, both the cellular and humoral systems appear to be involved in the disease process.

It is important to note that the effects of herbs on MS itself have never been specifically studied. Immune-stimulating effects have been observed in *scientific studies*, such as test tube experiments or animal studies. However, it is not clear how these observed effects translate into *human clinical studies*. In other words, it is not known whether a herb that produces an immune effect in a scientific study will necessarily cause any significant effect in a person with an immune system–related disease such as MS. It is also important to note that only a few scientific studies have been undertaken for some herb effects on the immune system. As a result, *much more research must be done* to more fully understand how these herbs affect immune function and how they might possibly affect MS disease activity.

Many commonly used herbs may stimulate the immune system (see Table 23.2). Echinacea is the most well known of these herbs. Some other herbs in this category are among the most popular herbs in the United States, including alfalfa, Asian ginseng, astragalus, cat's claw, garlic, saw palmetto, and Siberian ginseng. Other immune-stimulating herbs may be found in this book in the chapters on Asian herbal medicine and Ayurvedic medicine.

For people with MS, the use of one rather uncommon herb, woody nightshade stem, is specifically discouraged in *The German Commission E Monographs*, an authoritative text on herbal medicine [3]. It is not clear if

TABLE 23.2. *Herbs That May Stimulate the Immune System*

Alfalfa	Celandine	Licorice
Arnica	Drosera	Maitake mushroom
Astragalus	Echinacea	Mistletoe, European
Boneset	Garlic	Reishi mushroom
Calendula	Ginseng, Asian	Saw palmetto
Cat's claw	Ginseng, Siberian	Shiitake mushroom
		Stinging nettle

this recommendation is based on any possible immune effects of woody nightshade stem.

In some herbal therapy books, MS is correctly described as an immune disorder; however, it is then assumed that MS is caused by *too little* immune-system activity and that immune-stimulating herbs are beneficial. Consequently, some of the herbs in Table 23.2 often are *recommended* for MS.

MS is an immune disorder, but it is caused by *excessive* immune-system activity. Thus, on a theoretical basis, immune-stimulating herbs may worsen the disease.

It is impossible to develop strict guidelines about the use of these herbs because their exact effects on MS are not known. It may be best for people with MS to simply avoid these herbs. If they are used, they probably should not be used in high doses or on a long-term basis.

Sedating Herbs

Many herbs may produce sedation (Table 23.3). Some of the more common herbs on this list are Asian ginseng, chamomile, goldenseal, kava kava, St. John's wort, Siberian ginseng, and valerian.

The sedating effects of these herbs may occur when they are taken alone or in combination with sedating medication or alcohol. This is important because fatigue is common in MS. In addition, medications with possible sedating effects are used commonly in MS, including lioresal (Baclofen), tizanidine (Zanaflex), diazepam (Valium), and clonazepam (Klonopin).

Herbs to Avoid with Urinary Tract Infections

Some herbs may irritate the urinary tract (Table 23.4). The most commonly used herb on this list is coffee. The herbs in this category may worsen the

TABLE 23.3.   *Herbs with Possible Sedating Effects*

Balm	Ginseng, Asian	St. John's wort
Barberry	Ginseng, Siberian	Sage
Black cohosh	Goldenseal	Sassafras
Calamus	Gotu kola (hydrocotyle)	Scullcap
Calendula	Henbane	Shepherd's purse
California poppy	Hops	Stinging nettle
Capsicum (cayenne)	Jamaican dogwood	Valerian
Catnip	Kava kava	Wild carrot
Celery	Lavender	Wild lettuce
Chamomile	Lemon balm	Withania (ashwagandha)
Couchgrass	Motherwort	Yerba mansa
Elecampine	Passionflower	

TABLE 23.4. *Herbs That May Irritate the Urinary Tract*

Asiatic dogwood	Eucalyptus	Pine needles
Asparagus	Fragrant sumach	Rue
Buchu	Guarana	Sandalwood
Celery	Horseradish	Sassafras
Cinnamon	Juniper berries	Tea
Coffee	Lovage	Thyme
Cola nut	Maté	Watercress
Copaiba oleoresin	Myrrh gum	Yellow cedar
Cubeb	Parsley	Yerba mansa
Dill seed	Pennyroyal	

effects of UTIs, which occur frequently in some women with MS. In addition, frequent use or high doses of these herbs may irritate the urinary tract even when an infection does not exist (4).

Herbs That May Interact with Steroids

Steroids sometimes are used to treat MS attacks. Some herbs (Table 23.5) probably should be avoided with steroid use because they may worsen steroid side effects (increase blood sugar or decrease blood potassium) or increase the potency of the steroids. The more commonly used herbs on this list are Asian ginseng, ephedra (*ma huang*), licorice, and senna.

Herbs That May Interact with Antidepressant Medications

Tricyclic antidepressants are an older class of antidepressant medications. These drugs, which include amitriptyline (Elavil) and nortriptyline (Pamelor), may be used to treat depression or pain in people with MS. When using these antidepressants, one should avoid St. John's wort, belladonna, henbane, jimson weed, mandrake, and scopolia. St. John's wort also should be avoided when taking the antidepressants known as SSRIs, which include fluoxetine (Prozac), sertraline (Zoloft), and paroxetine (Paxil).

TABLE 23.5. *Herbs That May Interact with Steroids*

Aloe	Figwort
Bayberry	Ginseng, Asian
Buckthorn	Gotu kola (hydrocotyle)
Cascara sagrada	Licorice
Devil's claw	Lily-of-the-valley
Elecampine	Pheasant's eye
Ephedra (*ma huang*)	Senna
Fenugreek	Squill

Herbs That May Interact with Amantadine

Amantadine is used frequently in MS to treat fatigue. Confusion or sedation may occur if amantadine is taken along with belladonna, henbane, jimson weed, mandrake, or scopolia.

Herbs That May Interact with Interferons

Interferon medications (Avonex, Betaseron, Rebif) that are used to treat MS may cause liver toxicity. Similarly, some herbs may produce liver toxicity. The use of these herbs along with interferons may increase the risk of liver toxicity. Herbs with possible liver toxicity include alkanna, alpine ragwort, bishop's weed, black cohosh, boldo, borage seed oil, butterbur, chaparral, coltsfoot, comfrey, dusty miller, echinacea, eucalyptus, germander, golden ragwort, gotu kola, gravel root, greater celandine, ground ivy, groundsel, hemp agrimony, hound's tongue, kava kava, khella, pennyroyal oil, tansy ragwort, and red yeast.

Herbs That May Interact with Methotrexate

Methotrexate is a chemotherapy drug sometimes used to treat MS. It may produce adverse effects if taken with aspirin-like chemicals known as salicylates. Herbs that contain salicylates should be avoided when taking methotrexate. These include aspen, meadowsweet, poplar, sweet birch, willow, and wintergreen. Methotrexate may cause liver toxicity. This risk of liver toxicity may increase if methotrexate is take along with herbs that may have liver toxicity (see the section "Herbs That May Interact with Interferons").

Potentially Dangerous Herbs or Herbs with Unstudied Toxicity

Some herbs have been associated with significant toxic effects or have not been subjected to toxicity evaluations (Table 23.6). These herbs should be avoided. In spite of reports of toxicity, it is possible to purchase many of these herbs in the United States.

Potentially dangerous herbs that are sometimes specifically recommended for MS include borage seed oil, chaparral, comfrey, lobelia, and

TABLE 23.6. *Herbs with Potential Toxicity or Uninvestigated Toxicity*

Angelica	Dong-quai	Lobelia	Sage
Blue cohosh	Ephedra (*ma huang*)	Mistletoe	Sassafras
Borage	Foxglove	Muira puama	Scullcap
Calamus	Garcinia	Pangamic acid	Suma
Chaparral	Germander	Pau d'arco	Tansy
Coltsfoot	Kombucha	Pennyroyal	Wormwood
Comfrey	Life root	Rue	Yohimbe

yohimbe. Borage seed oil, chaparral, and comfrey may contain chemicals that are toxic to the liver. Lobelia may potentially cause a rapid heart rate, low blood pressure, seizures, coma, or death. As described previously, yohimbe may produce psychiatric problems, high blood pressure, and worsening of liver or kidney disease.

Another herb in this category, ephedra (*ma huang*), is claimed to be effective for fatigue and multiple other conditions. Ephedra use has been associated with severely increased blood pressure, abnormal heart rhythms, heart failure, and death. Also, ephedra may cause dizziness, irritability, headache, upset stomach, and heart palpitations. Due to these side effects, ephedra was banned for sale in the United States in April 2004.

Conclusion

Herbs should be used with caution by people with MS. Many herbs with no well-documented benefits may potentially worsen MS or interact with MS medications. Some herbs may be of benefit for specific MS-related symptoms. These include St. John's wort for depression, valerian for insomnia, cranberry for the prevention of UTIs, and psyllium for constipation.

Although some information is available about herbs and MS, much more remains to be learned, even for the well-studied herbs such as echinacea and St. John's wort. In a sense, the message for herbs and MS is similar to that for unconventional medicine and MS as a whole—some of the therapies may be beneficial, some may be harmful, and nearly all are not fully understood.

Additional Readings

Books

Blumenthal M, ed. *The Complete German Commission E Monographs: Therapeutic Guide to Herbal Medicines.* Austin: American Botanical Council, 1998.

Bowling AC, Stewart TS. *Dietary Supplements and Multiple Sclerosis: A Health Professional's Guide.* New York: Demos Medical Publishing, 2004.

Brinker F. *Herb Contraindications and Drug Interactions.* Oregon: Eclectic Medical Publishers, 1998.

Fetrow CW, Avila JR. *Professional's Handbook of Complementary and Alternative Medicines.* Philadelphia: Lippincott, Williams, & Wilkins, 2004.

Fragakis AS. *The Health Professional's Guide to Popular Dietary Supplements.* The American Dietetic Association, 2003.

Jellin JM, Batz F, Hitchens K, et al. *Natural Medicines Comprehensive Database.* Therapeutic Research Faculty, 2006.

Newall CA, Anderson LA, Phillipson JD. *Herbal Medicines: A Guide for Healthcare Professionals*. London: The Pharmaceutical Press, 1996.

Polman CH, Thompson AJ, Murray TJ, et al. *Multiple Sclerosis: The Guide to Treatment and Management*. New York: Demos Medical Publishing, 2006.

Schulz V, Hansel R, Tyler VE. *Rational Phytotherapy: A Physicians' Guide to Herbal Medicine*. Berlin: Springer-Verlag, 1998.

Ulbricht CE, Basch EM, eds. *Natural Standard Herb and Supplement Reference: Evidence-Based Clinical Reviews*. St. Louis: Elsevier-Mosby, 2005.

24

Hippotherapy and Therapeutic Horseback Riding

Hippotherapy is an unusual term that refers to the use of horseback riding for therapeutic effects. The word is derived from the Greek word *hippos*, which means horse. Therapeutic horseback riding, a technique related to hippotherapy, aims to both produce therapeutic effects and teach riding skills.

Horseback riding as a therapy has been used for thousands of years. It was used in Greece in the fifth century B.C. to rehabilitate injured soldiers. Hippocrates wrote of horseback riding as a "natural exercise." Similarly, wounded soldiers were treated with horseback riding in England during World War I.

More recently, Liz Hartel, a Danish woman who had polio, demonstrated the possible benefits of riding. She developed leg strength and coordination through riding, and eventually won a silver medal in dressage in the 1952 Olympic Games in Finland.

Riding therapy has been used since the 1940s in Europe, especially in Germany and Switzerland. Much of the published research in this area has been conducted in Germany. This type of therapy is a relative newcomer in the United States. The first center for therapeutic riding was established in Michigan, in 1969. More than 600 accredited therapeutic riding centers are now open in the United States.

Treatment Method

Hippotherapy and therapeutic riding often are done in conjunction with physical therapy. In riding therapy, a person is placed on a horse and monitored by a therapist, usually a trained physical therapist or occupational therapist. Typically, bareback pads are used, and straps or handholds are provided for stability. In addition to the conventional riding position, riders also may sit sideways, backwards, or even lie sideways or backwards. The person on the horse responds to the animal's movements with body movements. Unlike conventional horseback riding, in riding therapy, the rider does not attempt to control the horse. Rather, the therapist, who may be on the ground or on the horse with the rider, controls the horse and adjusts the treatment as indicated.

Studies in MS and Other Conditions

Hippotherapy is believed to be beneficial for people with walking difficulties because the rhythmic movements of the human pelvis while horseback riding are similar to those that occur with walking. In addition, the variations in the horse's speed, stride, and direction are thought to be beneficial for walking impairments. Some studies indicate that approximately 100 different horse movements are transmitted to the rider during each minute of riding. Some psychological benefits also may be related to developing a bond with the horse, developing relationships with the therapist and other riders, and simply being outdoors.

Although hippotherapy frequently is discussed in relation to multiple sclerosis (MS), only a few studies have specifically evaluated its possible benefits for people with this disease. A Swedish study evaluated the effects of hippotherapy on multiple symptoms in 11 people with MS (1). In this small study, ten people improved in at least one of the areas assessed. The most consistent improvement, found in ten people, was in balance. An improvement in emotional functioning was found in eight. Pain and the ability to perform daily activities improved in a few people. Muscle stiffness improved in only one person. It was noted that different people had different responses to hippotherapy—thus, it may be optimal to have an individualized approach to the therapy and to the expectations of the therapy.

Other smaller studies of hippotherapy in MS have been reported. A preliminary study, done in 1988, examined the effects of twice-weekly therapeutic riding for 9 weeks in people with MS (2). Riding was associated with improved walking and improved mood. In another study, reported in 1991, it was found that one person with MS had a more normal walking pattern after once-weekly riding for 4 weeks (3). Studies of hippotherapy indicate that it may have both physical and psychosocial benefits. One preliminary study in Pennsylvania was reported at an MS conference (Consortium of Multiple Sclerosis Centers) in May 1999. In this study, it was found that hippotherapy undertaken for 6 to 8 weeks improved balance and the quality of life in three people with MS.

Hippotherapy and therapeutic riding have been researched extensively in children with cerebral palsy. These studies are relevant to MS because people with cerebral palsy and MS experience some of the same neurologic difficulties, including walking unsteadiness, stiffness, and weakness.

Unfortunately, many of the studies on cerebral palsy have been small, poorly designed, and have not included a placebo group. In addition, inconsistent results have been obtained. In studies of once- or twice-weekly therapy, ranging from 8 to 26 weeks, therapy has been associated with improvement in walking, running, jumping, muscle strength, and muscle stiffness. In addition, one study found that children walked more efficiently and used less energy to walk after therapy. Improvement in standing and sitting postures also has been associated with hippotherapy in some studies.

Studies have been done on other conditions. In a German study of people with significant arm or leg weakness, hippotherapy improved stiffness (spasticity), urinary function, bowel function, mood, and sleep. One study of children with language disorders reported improvement in language skills and self-esteem.

Although some studies have reported positive effects in MS, cerebral palsy, and other conditions, the results of these studies are not conclusive. Clearly, better-designed studies using larger numbers of patients are needed to more fully understand the effects of this type of therapy.

Side Effects

The most obvious risk of hippotherapy and therapeutic horseback riding is falling from the horse. People with MS who are experiencing a significant exacerbation should probably avoid hippotherapy because they may be especially unstable. Also, riding may not be possible for people with difficulty sitting, decreased head control, and severe muscle stiffness or spasticity. People with severe fatigue or symptoms worsened by heat should be cautious about riding in hot weather. The American Hippotherapy Association lists a number of other conditions that should preclude hippotherapy, including severe osteoporosis, bone fractures, herniated disks, instability of the spine, severe arthritis, the use of anticoagulant medication, wounds or sores on weight-bearing surfaces, and seizures. The Association also recommends that therapy be done cautiously with some conditions, including diabetes, hip joint abnormalities, obesity, mild or moderate osteoporosis, allergies to dust or horsehair, heart disease, incontinence, and recent surgery.

Practical Information

It is best to receive hippotherapy from a qualified therapist who works at a riding center. For those with mild disability, therapeutic riding sessions provide the benefits of riding as well as riding lessons. When the riding skills are learned, riding may be done independently.

Sessions generally last 20 to 30 minutes. Fees are approximately $35 to $150 per hour. Health insurance may cover some of the cost of the therapy.

More information on hippotherapy and therapeutic horseback riding may be obtained from:

- The American Hippotherapy Association, North American Riding for the Handicapped Association (www.narha.org), P.O. Box 33150, Denver CO 80233 (800-369-RIDE)
- The National Center for Equine Facilitated Therapy (www.nceft.org), 5001 Woodside Road, Woodside CA 94062 (650-851-2271)

Conclusion

Hippotherapy and therapeutic horseback riding are low-risk, moderate-cost therapies that offer possible benefits for multiple MS-associated symptoms, including walking difficulties, spasticity, weakness, bladder and bowel problems, and depression. Further studies are needed to determine the effects of this therapy more definitively.

Additional Readings

Journal Articles

Bertoti DB. Effect of therapeutic horseback riding on posture in children with cerebral palsy. *Phys Ther* 1988;68:1505–1512.

Hammer A, Nilsagard Y, Forsberg A, et al. Evaluation of therapeutic riding (Sweden)/hippotherapy (United States). A single-subject experimental design study replicated in eleven patients with multiple sclerosis. *Physiother Theory Prac* 2005;1:51–77.

MacKinnon JR, Noh S, Lariviere J, et al. A study of therapeutic effects of horseback riding for children with cerebral palsy. *Phys Occup Ther Ped* 1995;15:17–31.

MacKinnon JR, Noh S, Laliberte D, et al. Therapeutic horseback riding: a review of the literature. *Phys Occup Ther Ped* 1995;15:1–15.

McGibbon NH, Andrade C-K, Widener G, et al. Effect of an equine-movement therapy program on gait, energy expenditure, and motor function in children with spastic cerebral palsy: a pilot study. *Dev Med Child Neurol* 1998;40:754–762.

Meregillano G. Hippotherapy. *Phys Med Rehabil Clin N Amer* 2004;15:843–854.

Pauw J. Therapeutic horseback riding studies: problems experienced by researchers. *Physiother* 2000;86:523–527.

25

Homeopathy

$\mathcal{H}$omeopathy is one of the more controversial forms of complementary and alternative medicine (CAM). Much of the controversy is due to the fact that the basic principles of homeopathy are in conflict with many of the fundamental concepts of conventional medicine as well as those of chemistry, biology, and physics. In spite of these controversial ideas, homeopathy is, on a worldwide basis, one of the most popular forms of CAM.

Homeopathy is a system of medicine that was developed in the 1800s by Samuel Hahnemann, a German physician. Homeopathy was very popular in Europe and North America in the nineteenth century. The use of homeopathy in the United States declined from the 1950s to the 1970s, but its popularity has rebounded since.

Homeopathy is used globally. On a worldwide basis, $1 billion to $5 billion are spent yearly on this form of treatment. Homeopathy is most popular in Europe and India. Homeopathic remedies are dispensed in pharmacies in France. In the United States, more than $150 million are spent annually on homeopathic remedies, and approximately 1 percent of American adults currently use homeopathy.

Treatment Method

Homeopathy is based on several principles. One is the "law of similars," which states that "like cures like." Variations of this principle have been used in other forms of medicine for thousands of years. In homeopathy, it is believed that, if large doses of a substance produce specific symptoms, very small doses of that substance will cure the same symptoms. For example, because large doses of arsenic produce stomach cramps, very low doses of arsenic may be used to treat them.

The use of very low doses of substances is another important principle of homeopathy. Natural substances, such as herbs, minerals, or animal

150

products, are mixed with water or alcohol and then diluted 1:10 or 1:100. These dilutions are then repeated many times, so that the final solution is *extremely dilute*. In homeopathic notation, *X* is used for 1:10 dilutions, *C* is used for 1:100 dilutions, and a number is used for the number of times a specific dilution is made. For example, *12X* refers to a solution that has been diluted 12 times in a 1:10 manner, and *30C* signifies a 1:100 dilution performed 30 times.

Many homeopathic preparations are so dilute that they do not contain even a single molecule of the original substance. In this situation, it is argued that the water has a "memory" for the substance that it once contained. Also, by the laws of homeopathy, it is believed that a solution is more potent if it contains less of a substance. These ideas of water "memory" and increased potency with increased dilution, which defy the conventional laws of physics, chemistry, and biology, generate much of the controversy about homeopathy. The use of these dilute solutions has raised questions about whether homeopathy is simply a way to produce a placebo response.

Homeopathy is focused on identifying both symptoms and the personal features of the patient. In addition, homeopathic treatment aims to use the body's natural healing processes. This is in contrast to conventional medicine, in which symptoms are used primarily to diagnose an underlying disease; the personal characteristics of an individual are not a critical component of the diagnostic process or choice of therapy, and treatment involves the use of drugs and other therapies that improve the disease process but do not necessarily alter the body's natural healing abilities.

Because of the detailed evaluation process, homeopaths probably become more familiar with their patients and spend more time with them than do physicians who practice conventional medicine. One study found that physicians in the United States who practice homeopathy spend more than twice as much time with their patients than do physicians who do not practice homeopathy. The in-depth relationship that develops in homeopathy may be important for the healing process and may certainly augment any type of placebo effect.

A variety of homeopathic remedies has been suggested for multiple sclerosis (MS). The treatment regimen depends on the individual and the specific symptoms. Homeopathic remedies sometimes recommended for MS include *Argentum nitricum, Aurum muriaticum, and Plumbum metallicum.*

Could Homeopathy Be a Placebo Effect?

Because the approach of a homeopath may be conducive to a placebo effect and because homeopathic remedies may not actually contain any active substance, much of the beneficial effect of homeopathy may be a placebo response. Even if it is a placebo response, it may be helpful in certain situations. It is known that placebos are generally 30 to 40 percent effective. For situations in which conventional medicine has no particularly effective therapy, homeopathy may be a way to provide at least a placebo response. Jeremy Swayne, an English homeopath, writes: "If homeopathy is placebo, it presents us with a rich and systematic study of the working of the placebo response, which fully deserves to be taken seriously and investigated. If it is not, then the implications are even more startling" (1).

Different Homeopathic Approaches

Homeopathy includes both classic and nonclassic approaches. The classic approach involves a detailed evaluation of the patient by a practitioner who develops a personalized treatment plan on the basis of the clinical evaluation. In contrast, the nonclassic approach does not involve a homeopath. Instead, a certain condition is identified, and treatment for that condition is then given. In the nonclassic approach, the condition may be identified by the affected individual or by a non-homeopath practitioner who uses homeopathic therapy.

Studies in MS and Other Conditions

Whether homeopathic therapy produces effects that are greater than those produced by placebos is subject to controversy. Many clinical studies have evaluated homeopathic treatment for a variety of conditions. Unfortunately, many of these studies have been poorly conducted, and the results often are not conclusive.

To attempt to clarify this area, two recent studies have evaluated the results of multiple homeopathic studies. In 1991, a report examined 107 homeopathic studies published between 1966 and 1990 (2). Most of the studies were of low quality. However, approximately three-fourths of them reported beneficial effects. A research article in 1997 analyzed the results of 89 homeopathic studies (3). This study concluded that no studies have clearly proved homeopathy to be an effective therapy for any specific condition. However, it also was argued in this study that the effects of homeopathy are not simply placebo effects. A subsequent and more detailed analysis of the same data led to the conclusion that more rigorous studies yield less positive results (4). A 2005 study evaluated multiple homeopathic and conventional medicine clinical trials (5). Overall, the quality of the homeopathy trials was higher than that of the conventional medicine trials. When large trials of high quality were examined, it was found that homeopathy generally produced a much weaker treatment effect than did conventional medicine. The authors of the study concluded that these results were consistent with the concept that the clinical effects of homeopathy are placebo effects.

Homeopathy is not one of the more commonly used forms of CAM among people with MS in the United States. In contrast, homeopathy appears to be used frequently by people with MS in Europe. Studies have shown that, among people with MS, homeopathy is the most popular form of CAM in Holland and one of the most popular CAM therapies in Germany.

Specific homeopathic remedies sometimes are recommended for MS. The medical literature contains isolated reports (anecdotes) of individuals with MS treated with homeopathy. However, no well-documented large studies have investigated the effect of homeopathic treatment on MS.

Homeopathy has produced mixed results for neurologic diseases other than MS. Variable results or limited evidence for a therapeutic effect have been observed in studies of migraine, pain, and vertigo.

Viral infections, such as the common cold and flu, may lead to MS attacks. As a result, it may be helpful for people with MS to try to prevent viral infections or to shorten the time that they are affected by a viral infection. Limited options are available for the treatment or prevention of viral infections; these include simple preventive measures (such as hand-washing and avoiding exposure to infected people), the flu vaccination, and recently developed prescription medications that decrease the duration and severity of the flu. Supplements of unproven effectiveness for the common cold (echinacea, garlic, zinc, vitamin C) pose a theoretical risk for people with MS because of possible immune-stimulating activity.

Given the limited options, some people consider the use of homeopathy for preventing or treating viral infections. Studies of homeopathic therapies for viral syndromes have produced mixed results. Although homeopathy does not appear to be effective for flu prevention, positive results have been obtained in some studies of flu treatment. For people with an interest in homeopathic remedies, this approach may be a reasonable possibility for the treatment of viral infections. If homeopathy is used, available conventional therapies should be discussed with a physician, and it must be kept in mind that the homeopathic therapies are not proven to be effective.

Side Effects

Overall, homeopathy is very well tolerated. Homeopathy should not be used in lieu of conventional medical therapy. Some of the substances used in homeopathy, such as snake venom, arsenic, and poison oak, are potentially toxic. However, the doses of these substances are generally so low that they do not cause problems.

Homeopaths note several precautions that should be taken. One is that treatment should be discontinued when a symptom resolves. Otherwise, the treatment may produce recurrence of the symptom. Also, *antidotes* may interfere with treatment. Antidotes include coffee, acupuncture, x-rays, and dental drilling. Finally, a person receiving homeopathic treatment should notify the homeopath of any conventional medical treatment being used, because this information may affect the homeopathic interpretation of symptoms.

Practical Information

Initial visits with a homeopath are typically 60 minutes in length and cost between $100 and $140. Follow-up visits are 20 to 30 minutes and cost about $60.

More information on homeopathy can be obtained from:

- The Council on Homeopathic Education (www.chedu.org), 13 Duchess Terrace, Beacon NY 12508 (703-229-4343)
- The National Center for Homeopathy (NCH) (www.homeopathic.org), 801 North Fairfax Street, Suite 306, Alexandria VA 22314 (877-624-0613 or 703-548-7790)

Conclusion

Homeopathy is a low-risk, low- to moderate-cost therapy with unproven effectiveness. No rigorous studies have specifically evaluated the effect of homeopathy on MS. For people with MS who are interested in this approach, it may be worth considering for mild conditions (such as viral infections or mild MS-related symptoms) or for conditions for which conventional medical therapy is ineffective or only partially effective. Homeopathy should not be used in place of conventional medicine. Specifically, homeopathic treatment should not be used for controlling MS disease activity in place of conventional medications, such as glatiramer acetate (Copaxone), interferons (Avonex, Betaseron, Rebif), mitoxantrone (Novantrone), or natalizumab (Tysabri).

Additional Readings

Books

Chapman EH. Homeopathy. In: Weintraub MI, Micozzi MS, eds. *Alternative and Complementary Treatments in Neurologic Illness.* New York: Churchill Livingstone, 2001, pp. 51–67.

Ernst E, ed. *The Desktop Guide to Complementary and Alternative Medicine: An Evidence-Based Approach.* Edinburgh: Mosby. 2001, pp. 53–55.

Shinto L, Calabrese C. Naturopathic medicine in neurological disorders. In: Oken BS, ed. *Complementary Therapies in Neurology.* London: Parthenon Publishing, 2004, pp. 136–138.

Swayne J. *Homeopathic Method: Implications for Clinical Practice and Medical Science.* New York: Churchill Livingstone, 1998.

Journal Articles

Jonas WB, Kaptchuk TJ, Linde K. A critical overview of homeopathy. *Annals Int Med* 2003;138:393–399.

Kleijnen J, Knipschild P, ter Riet G. Clinical trials of homoeopathy. *Br Med J* 1991;302:316–326.

Linde K, Clausius N, Ramirez G, et al. Are the clinical effects of homoeopathy placebo effects? A meta-analysis of placebo-controlled trials. *Lancet* 1997; 350:834–843.

Linde K, Scholz M, Ramirez G, et al. Impact of study quality on outcome in placebo-controlled trials of homeopathy. *J Clin Epidemiol* 1999;52:631–636.

Shang A, Huwiler-Muntener K, Nartey L, et al. Are the clinical effects of homeopathy placebo effects? Comparative study of placebo-controlled trials of homeopathy and allopathy. *Lancet* 2005;366:726–732.

Whitmarsh TE. Homeopathy in multiple sclerosis. *Complement Ther Nurs Midwifery* 2003;9:5–9.

26

Hyperbaric Oxygen

Hyperbaric oxygen treatment is a form of oxygen therapy. It is claimed to be an effective treatment for a large number of diseases, including multiple sclerosis (MS). Unfortunately, many of the claims about this therapy are not supported by research evidence.

Treatment Method

In this type of treatment, a person breathes oxygen under increased pressure in a specially designed chamber. The procedure increases the oxygen content of the blood and thereby increases the amount of oxygen in different body tissues. The increased oxygen level in the blood and tissues is believed to be helpful for a variety of medical conditions.

Studies in MS and Other Conditions

The original study that generated interest in hyperbaric oxygen and MS was published in the prestigious *New England Journal of Medicine* in 1983 (1). In this study of 17 people with MS, 12 showed improvement and 5 had long-lasting improvement. In addition to this clinical study, animal studies have produced positive results. In animals, hyperbaric oxygen protects against experimental allergic encephalomyelitis (EAE), an experimental form of MS.

Advocates of hyperbaric oxygen therapy for MS cite the positive clinical study from 1983. However, seven studies performed after the 1983 study did *not* demonstrate any consistent therapeutic effect for hyperbaric oxygen. In a few studies, a mild improvement in bladder problems was noted. A 1995 review of hyperbaric oxygen treatment trials in MS concluded that hyperbaric oxygen did not produce significant benefits in MS and that this therapy should not be used for MS (2). Another analysis of hyperbaric oxygen trials in MS, published in 2004, concluded that this therapy did not produce consistent evidence for a therapeutic effect, should not be used on a routine basis, and should not be investigated further in MS (3). The methodology and the interpretation of the results of past trials of hyperbaric oxygen in MS have been criticized (4).

Hyperbaric oxygen is an accepted therapy for a limited number of specific medical conditions. For example, it is an effective treatment for burns and severe infections. Other rare uses included decompression sickness (as a result of deep-sea diving), carbon monoxide poisoning, air bubbles in the blood stream caused by medical procedures, and tissue injury caused by radiation exposure.

Side Effects

In general, hyperbaric oxygen is well tolerated. Mild and reversible visual changes may sometimes occur. Rarely, more serious side effects may occur, including seizures, pressure injury to the ear, cataracts, and collapsed lungs.

Practical Information

Hyperbaric oxygen therapy is time-consuming and expensive. Each session lasts for 1 to 5 hours, and a course of therapy may require 20 sessions. Individual sessions cost between $75 and $300. A course of treatment may cost several thousand dollars. Hyperbaric oxygen therapy is costly because the equipment is expensive, technicians monitor the equipment during therapy, and many treatment sessions usually are involved.

Conclusion

No consistent evidence supports the use of hyperbaric oxygen therapy in MS. Multiple clinical trials and reviews of these trials have concluded that it is not an effective treatment for MS. In addition, it may be very expensive, requires much time and effort, and occasionally produces serious side effects.

Additional Readings

Journal Articles

Bennett M, Heard R. Hyperbaric oxygen therapy for multiple sclerosis. *Cochrane Database Syst Rev* 2004;(1):CD003057.

Kleijnen J, Knipschild P. Hyperbaric oxygen for multiple sclerosis: review of controlled trials. *Acta Neurol Scand* 1995;91:330–334.

Tibbles PM, Edelsberg JS. Hyperbaric oxygen therapy. *N Engl J Med* 1996;334: 1642–1648.

27

Hypnosis

*H*ypnosis uses mental processes to alter physical processes. In this way, hypnosis, like biofeedback and meditation, is a type of mind–body therapy.

Medical interest in hypnosis has existed for hundreds of years. In the late 1700s, Franz Mesmer, an Austrian physician, used calming gestures and words to relax patients and, presumably, balance their magnetic energy. A commission appointed by the French Academy criticized this technique, known as *mesmerism*, and Mesmer was claimed to be a fraud. More recently, a magical, evil, mind-controlling view of hypnosis was promoted by vaudeville performers and magicians.

Hypnosis has gained some acceptance by conventional medicine despite these negative representations of the technique. It was deemed a valid medical treatment in England in 1955 and in the United States in 1958. Research studies support the use of hypnosis for some conditions. However, many physicians and other mainstream health care professionals do not readily incorporate hypnosis into their medical practices.

Treatment Method

In hypnosis, an individual enters a trancelike state. In this state of focused concentration, which is generally produced by a hypnotherapist, an individual is particularly vulnerable to suggestion. As a result, during hypnosis, a therapist makes suggestions of therapeutic value. For example, anxiety may be improved with suggestions for relaxation, and pain may be relieved with suggestions for numbness. In self-hypnosis, individuals make specific suggestions themselves. Self-hypnosis usually is most effective when it is taught by a trained therapist.

There is great variability in the success of hypnosis. Some of this variability is due to the fact that different people have different degrees of susceptibility to hypnotic suggestion. Approximately two-thirds of the population are moderately susceptible to suggestion, and 5 to 10 percent of people are extremely susceptible. Children and young adults are especially responsive to hypnosis.

Studies in MS and Other Conditions

No large studies have specifically evaluated the possible benefits of hypnosis for multiple sclerosis (MS). Published *case reports* describe the response of individuals with MS to hypnosis (1,2). In these reports, improvement is noted in multiple MS-related symptoms. There is also a study of the effects of *autogenic training*, a technique similar to hypnosis, on 22 people with MS (3). Autogenic training involves mental exercises using relaxation and suggestion. It is aimed at teaching people to recognize the origin of certain physical and mental disorders and use that awareness for self-treatment. In the study of MS, autogenic training was associated with increased energy and less limitation in roles due to physical and emotional difficulties.

Symptoms that may occur with MS have been investigated in people with other conditions. Anxiety, which occurs frequently in MS, may be reduced through hypnosis-induced relaxation. Also, hypnosis may be an effective therapy for pain, which may be a particularly bothersome symptom in MS. Hypnosis appears to relieve different types of pain, including headache and pain associated with surgery, cancer, and fibromyalgia, a rheumatologic condition. Hypnosis may be used during surgery to reduce the amount of anesthesia or to completely eliminate the need for anesthesia in some cases. Hypnosis also may be beneficial for insomnia. Among other neurologic disorders, some beneficial effects of hypnosis have been reported in people with strokes, head injury, and spinal cord injury.

The effects of hypnosis on immune-system function have been investigated in limited studies. Mixed results have been obtained in studies of immune-function changes associated with hypnosis-induced relaxation. Hypnotic suggestions may be made to attempt to specifically alter immune function. In one study, four hypnotized individuals were given the suggestion to decrease their immunologic response to a skin test for tuberculosis; all of them inhibited this reaction. Overall, however, the studies in this area have limitations, and further research is needed to determine if hypnosis produces immunologic changes that are significant enough to affect disease processes.

Side Effects

Hypnosis usually is safe. Although some movies and television shows portray hypnotized individuals performing evil tasks, this is not an accurate view. People cannot be forced into hypnosis, and hypnotized people cannot be unwittingly instructed to commit undesirable acts. People with psychiatric disorders may experience adverse effects and should discuss their situation with a psychiatrist before considering hypnosis.

Practical Information

Hypnotherapy sessions are generally 30 to 90 minutes in length and cost between $60 and $150. An average course of treatment involves 6 to 12 weekly sessions. Several organizations provide information about hypnosis:

- The American Society of Clinical Hypnosis (www.asch.net), 140 North Bloomingdale Road, Bloomingdale IL 60018-4740 (630-980-4740)
- Society for Clinical and Experimental Hypnosis (www.sceh.us), 221 Rivermoor St., Boston MA 02132 (617-469-1981)

Some health insurance companies reimburse for hypnosis.

Conclusion

Hypnosis is a well-tolerated, low- to moderate-cost therapy. Hypnosis may relieve some MS-associated symptoms, including pain, anxiety, and insomnia.

Additional Readings

Books

Cassileth BR. *The Alternative Medicine Handbook*. New York: W.W. Norton, 1998:122–130.

Benham G, Nash MR. Hypnosis. In: Oken BS, ed. *Complementary Therapies in Neurology*. London: Parthenon Publishing, 2004, pp. 169–187.

Ernst E, ed. *The Desktop Guide to Complementary and Alternative Medicine: An Evidence-Based Approach*. Edinburgh: Mosby, 2001, pp. 56–58.

Hammond DC, Kabbani S. Neurohypnosis. In: Weintraub MI, Micozzi MS, eds. *Alternative and Complementary Treatments in Neurologic Illness*. New York: Churchill Livingstone, 2001, pp. 287–295.

Spencer JW, Jacobs JJ. *Complementary and Alternative Medicine: An Evidence-Based Approach*. St. Louis: Mosby, 2003.

Journal Articles

Dane JR. Hypnosis for pain and neuromuscular rehabilitation with multiple sclerosis: case summary, literature review, and analysis of outcomes. *Int J Clin Exp Hypn* 1996;44:208–231.

Hall H, Minnes L, Olness K. The psychophysiology of voluntary immunomodulation. *Int J Neurosci* 1993;69:221–234.

Miller GE, Cohen S. Psychological interventions and the immune system: a meta-analytic review and critique. *Health Psychol* 2001;20:47–63.

Smith GR, McKenzie JM, Marmer DJ, et al. Psychologic modulation of the human immune response to *Varicella zoster. Arch Intern Med* 1985;145:221–235.

Sutcher H. Hypnosis as adjunctive therapy for multiple sclerosis: a progress report. *Am J Clin Hypn* 1997;39:283–290.

Sutherland G, Andersen MB, Morris T. Relaxation and health-related quality of life in multiple sclerosis: the example of autogenic training. *J Behav Med* 2005; 28:249–256.

28

Low-Dose Naltrexone (LDN)

Naltrexone is an oral medication approved by the U.S. Food and Drug Administration (FDA) for the treatment of opiate and alcohol addiction. It has been proposed that low-dose naltrexone (LDN) is effective in preventing multiple sclerosis (MS) attacks, slowing the progression of MS, and treating MS symptoms. LDN is claimed to be effective for multiple other diseases, including cancer, AIDS, rheumatoid arthritis, and Crohn disease. Dr. Bernard Bihari, a physician in New York City, was the first to propose that LDN may be an effective treatment for MS and other diseases. A patent for the use of naltrexone in MS has been awarded by the U.S. Patent Office.

Treatment Method

Naltrexone typically is used in oral doses of 50 milligrams daily. LDN treatment uses oral daily doses of 1.5 to 4.5 milligrams daily.

Studies in MS and Other Conditions

Many anecdotal reports exist of LDN providing beneficial effects in people with MS. Some of these anecdotal responses may be viewed on LDN-related websites:

- LDNers organization, www.LDNers.org
- The LDN Research Trust, www.ldnresearchtrust.org
- Remedy Find, www.remedyfind.org
- Low Dose Naltrexone organization, www.lowdosenaltrexone.org.

No published studies exist of LDN treatment in MS or in the animal model of MS.

Multiple theories have been proposed about mechanisms by which LDN could exert therapeutic effects in MS. It is claimed that LDN may produce immune changes that would be beneficial for MS. According to another theory, LDN decreases the formation of harmful chemicals known as free radicals, which then decreases *excitotoxicity*, a biochemical process that injures nerve cells (1).

Side Effects

In MS and other conditions, the safety of LDN use, especially on a long-term basis, is not known. Anecdotally, it has been reported that LDN may increase muscle stiffness and increase wakefulness (1).

Practical Information

Due to limited information about LDN, its use should be discussed with a health professional. It is not known if LDN affects the disease course in MS. As a result, LDN should not be used *instead* of conventional disease-modifying medications, such as interferons (Avonex, Betaseron, Rebif), glatiramer acetate (Copaxone), mitoxantrone (Novantrone), and natalizumab (Tysabri).

Conclusion

Many anecdotal reports exist of LDN producing beneficial effects in people with MS. No published clinical trials have evaluated the safety and effectiveness of LDN in MS. Further studies of LDN are needed, including human and animal studies of possible immune changes with the use of LDN and studies of the safety and effectiveness of LDN in the animal model of MS and in people with MS.

Additional Readings

Journal Articles

Agrawal YP. Low dose naltrexone therapy in multiple sclerosis. *Med Hypotheses* 2005;64:721–724.

29

Magnets and Electromagnetic Therapy

The use of magnets and electromagnetic fields is a type of *energy medicine*. Magnets and electricity have been used for medicinal purposes for thousands of years. They were used in ancient China to stimulate acupuncture sites. In the eleventh and twelfth centuries, it was claimed that lodestones, minerals with natural magnetic qualities, relieved a variety of medical conditions. Paracelsus, a sixteenth-century Swiss physician and alchemist, used magnets to treat seizures. In the eighteenth century, Franz Mesmer, an Austrian physician, proposed a theory of *animal magnetism* and wrote a book on the subject, *On the Medicinal Uses of the Magnet*. It was later found that his therapy was based on hypnotism (see the chapter on "Hypnosis"), not on any therapeutic effects of magnets. A large number of magnetic and electrical devices were promoted during the nineteenth century, which is sometimes referred to as the *golden age of medical electricity*. These devices included magnetic insoles, belts, girdles, and caps. The manufacture and sale of magnetic devices in the United States is now limited by the Food, Drug, and Cosmetic Act and the Medical Devices Amendment of 1976. Several recent research studies on magnets have increased interest in this type of therapy.

Treatment Method

Magnets and electricity are used in both conventional and unconventional medicine. In conventional medicine, small amounts of electrical energy produced by the body are measured for diagnostic reasons. For example, an electroencephalogram (EEG) records the electrical energy produced by the brain, whereas an electrocardiogram (ECG or EKG) detects electrical currents produced by the heart. Magnetic resonance imaging (MRI) machines use very powerful magnets to produce images of different parts of the body.

A unique therapeutic use of electrical energy has been employed recently to treat tremors in people with multiple sclerosis (MS), Parkinson's disease, and other neurologic disorders. In this treatment, an electrode is implanted in a brain region that controls body movements. Electrical stimulation of the electrode may significantly improve the tremor.

Magnets and electricity have many unconventional uses. Two types of electromagnetic therapy usually are considered for MS. One type of therapy, known as static magnetic therapy, uses magnets that are available as bracelets, belts, and even large mats that may be placed on a bed. The other form of therapy, known as pulsed electromagnetic field therapy, uses devices that produce pulsing magnetic fields at a specific frequency. The pulsing magnetic fields usually are weak, but some studies have used strong fields.

Multiple hypotheses exist about how magnets could produce therapeutic effects. For strong magnets placed on the spine, it has been proposed that the magnetic field alters nerve activity in the spinal cord in such a way that it decreases muscle stiffness. For weaker magnetic devices, it is often claimed that they correct disease-causing electrical imbalances in the body. For devices placed on acupuncture points, it is proposed that acupuncture-like effects occur, such as increases in the release of pain-relieving chemicals (opioids) in the body. Multiple other mechanisms have been proposed, including an alteration of the flow of electrically charged atoms (such as calcium) and changes in hormone levels and immune-system function.

Studies in MS and Other Conditions

Four placebo-controlled clinical studies of pulsed electromagnetic therapy in MS have been published. Three of these were conducted using weak electromagnetic fields, whereas one used strong fields applied to the spine. The study using strong fields was reported by a Danish group in 1996 (1). In 38 people with MS, it was found that the electromagnetic treatment was associated with a decrease in spasticity, compared with those who received sham therapy.

For studies using weak electromagnetic fields, variable results have been reported:

■   A promising two-part study of electromagnetic therapy in people with MS was reported from Hungary in 1987 (2). In the first part of this study, which included the use of a placebo therapy, 70 to 80 percent of the 20 treated participants benefited from pulsed electromagnetic therapy applied to the spine and legs. Spasticity, pain, and bladder function improved. In the second part of the investigation, electromagnetic treatment was used in 104 people in a less rigorous manner. Once again, symptoms improved in approximately 80 percent of people.

■ In 1997, a placebo-controlled study from the University of Washington examined the effects of a pulsing device applied to three acupuncture points on 30 people with MS (3). Benefits were noted with spasticity, bladder function, cognitive problems, fatigue, mobility, and vision.

■ In 2003, another placebo-controlled study treated 117 people with MS with a pulsing device placed on an acupuncture point near the shoulder (4). Beneficial effects were noted for fatigue and overall quality of life. No therapeutic effect for bladder function was noted. Variable results were obtained with spasticity.

Due to the variable findings and the lack of rigor in some of these clinical trials, further research is needed to determine whether this therapy has definite therapeutic effects in MS.

In addition to these studies of large groups of people with MS, reports exist of individuals with MS who experienced improvement in multiple symptoms using electromagnetic therapy. These reports are difficult to interpret because each study involved only a single person with MS.

Magnets have been investigated in other conditions. Among neurologic disorders, small studies have found that magnet therapy may be beneficial for people with pain associated with the delayed effects of polio (post-polio syndrome) and for people with pain resulting from nerve injury related to diabetes and other conditions. Variable results have been obtained in studies of magnet therapy for low back and neck pain.

Pulsing electromagnetic therapy may have multiple applications. This type of therapy stimulates the healing of bone fractures. It also may decrease swelling resulting from ankle sprains, promote healing of bedsores, and improve joint mobility and pain in people with arthritis.

Magnets are not approved by the U.S. Food and Drug Administration (FDA) for any medical condition at this time. However, pulsing devices are approved by the FDA for the treatment of bone fractures that do not heal.

A fascinating area of research involves applying pulsing high-intensity magnetic fields to the scalp. This technique, known as transcranial magnetic stimulation, takes advantage of the ability of magnetic fields to pass through bone. In this procedure, a very strong magnetic field applied to the scalp passes through the skull and stimulates the underlying brain tissue.

For example, applying magnetic stimulation to the region of the brain that controls movement results in movement of the corresponding part of the body. Some studies indicate that this therapy may be effective for multiple conditions, including depression and pain. Further studies are needed to determine the effectiveness and long-term safety of this technique. This approach is only available in designated research centers because very strong magnetic fields are used.

Side Effects

The use of magnets and pulsing electromagnetic fields is generally well tolerated, but the long-term safety of these therapies is not known. Women who are pregnant and people with pacemakers and other implanted electronic medical devices should consult a physician before using this type of therapy. When using one of the pulsing devices with a weak field, warnings are given that it should not be used by those with epilepsy, cancer, diabetes, or heart or kidney disease. High-intensity magnetic fields may have significant side effects (headaches, hearing loss, seizures, and other possible unknown effects) and should only be used under the direction of qualified clinical investigators.

Practical Information

A large number of magnets and pulsing electromagnetic devices are available. These vary greatly in terms of strength, size, shape, composition, and cost. Although some companies claim that their products are better because they produce a stronger electromagnetic field, it is not clear that a stronger field necessarily provides more benefit.

Conclusion

The use of low-intensity magnets and pulsing electromagnetic fields is usually well tolerated. Several studies suggest that pulsing electromagnetic fields may improve multiple MS symptoms, especially spasticity. Other symptoms that may benefit from this therapy are fatigue, pain, cognitive problems, bladder function, and walking difficulties. Further studies are required to determine definitively whether electromagnetic therapy in MS is effective and safe.

Additional Readings

Books

Cassileth BR. *The Alternative Medicine Handbook*. New York: W.W. Norton, 1998, pp. 299–304.

Oken BS, ed. *Complementary Therapies in Neurology*. London: Parthenon Publishing, 2004.

Polman CH, Thompson AJ, Murray TJ, et al. *Multiple Sclerosis: The Guide to Treatment and Management*. New York: Demos Medical Publishing, 2006, pp. 157–159.

Weintraub MI. Magnetic biostimulation in neurologic illness. In: Weintraub MI, Micozzi MS, eds. *Alternative and Complementary Treatments in Neurologic Iillness*. New York: Churchill Livingstone, 2001, pp. 278–286.

Journal Articles

Guseo A. Pulsing electromagnetic field therapy of multiple sclerosis by the Gyuling-Bordas device: double-blind, cross-over and open studies. *J Bioelec* 1987;6:23–35.

Nielsen JF, Sinkjaer T, Jakobsen J. Treatment of spasticity with repetitive magnetic stimulation: a double-blind placebo-controlled study. *Mult Scler* 1996; 2:227–232.

George MS, Lisanby SAH, Sackeim HA. Transcranial magnetic stimulation: applications in neuropsychiatry. *Arch Gen Psych* 1999;56:300–311.

Lappin MS, Lawrie FW, Richards TL, et al. Effects of a pulsed electromagnetic therapy on multiple sclerosis fatigue and quality of life: a double-blind, placebo controlled trial. *Alt Ther* 2003;9:38–48.

Richards TL, Lappin MS, Acosta-Urquidi J, et al. Double-blind study of pulsing magnetic field effects on multiple sclerosis. *J Alt Complem Med* 1997; 3:21–29.

Vallbona C, Hazlewood CF, Jurida G. Response of pain to static magnetic fields in postpolio patients: a double-blind pilot study. *Arch Phys Med Rehabil* 1997; 78:1200–1203.

30

Marijuana

*M*arijuana is derived from the plant known as *Cannabis sativa*, one of the oldest cultivated plants. It was grown in China nearly 5,000 years ago, and it has been used medicinally in many different cultures for thousands of years.

Treatment Method

Marijuana is available in several forms. The main active constituent in marijuana, a chemical known as delta-9-tetrahydrocannabinol or THC, is available by prescription as a pill (dronabinol or Marinol). Sativex, an oral spray that contains THC and another marijuana constituent, cannabidiol, is available by prescription in Canada. A synthetic form of THC (nabilone or Cesamet) also is available as a pill in Canada, Europe, and Australia. Most simply, the leaf may be smoked or eaten. The resin of the plant, hashish, also may be smoked.

Studies in MS and Other Conditions

The biologic effects of the chemicals in marijuana, known as *cannabinoids*, have been extensively investigated. These chemicals bind to proteins in the central nervous system (CNS) that decrease nerve cell activity. These proteins are known as *CB1 receptors*. Theoretically, binding to CB1 receptors could decrease some multiple sclerosis (MS)-associated symptoms, such as pain and spasticity. Also, cannabinoids bind to another type of protein known as *CB2 receptors*. Binding to these proteins, which are present on immune cells, may mildly suppress the immune system and could thus potentially slow down the disease course in MS. Other effects of cannabinoids, including antioxidant properties and inhibitory effects on a harmful process known as *excitotoxicity*, could also theoretically be beneficial for MS.

The effects of marijuana, THC, and nabilone have been studied in many diseases, including MS. Some of the recent interest in marijuana was generated by a 1999 report by the National Academy of Sciences/Institute of Medicine (NAS/IOM) that analyzed the scientific and clinical literature on the potential therapeutic effects of marijuana. The NAS/IOM report concluded that marijuana or THC may be effective in the treatment of pain, nausea associated with chemotherapy, and weight loss associated with AIDS and cancer. The report also cautioned against the long-term use of smoked marijuana, indicated that effective prescription medications are available for many conditions treated with marijuana, and suggested that methods of taking the drug, other than smoking it, should be developed.

The NAS/IOM analysis indicated that there have been some positive studies of marijuana and THC in relieving the spasticity or muscle stiffness associated with MS. These studies generally have been of mixed quality in that they have involved small numbers of patients (sometimes only one patient) and have not been well-designed clinical trials. Despite these limitations, promising reports have been published of marijuana, THC, or nabilone decreasing spasticity. These previous studies did not compare this treatment effect with that of prescription drugs for spasticity.

The first large formal clinical trial of marijuana in MS was conducted in the United Kingdom by Dr. John Zajicek and others (1). The initial results of this study, known as the CAMS (cannabinoids in MS) trial, were published in 2003. In this trial, more than 600 people with MS were treated for 13 weeks with oral THC, an extract of marijuana, or placebo. For several MS symptoms, objective testing by clinicians did not demonstrate any therapeutic effect for oral THC or marijuana extract. However, by subjective measures, which are based on the reporting of individuals in the study, beneficial effects were noted for marijuana extract and oral THC on spasticity, pain, and sleep quality. In a 12-month follow-up to this study, THC showed a small therapeutic effect on spasticity (2). Suggestive evidence was noted for a THC effect on disability. On the basis of these reports and other studies, a long-term clinical trial will be conducted in the United Kingdom. This study, known as CUPID (Cannaboid Use in Progressive Inflammatory Brain Disease), will evaluate the effects of oral THC on 500 people with MS over 3 years.

Multiple other studies have been undertaken of the use of marijuana or marijuana-derived chemicals in people with MS. An oral spray, Sativex, that contains marijuana-derived chemicals has been reported to improve spasticity (3)—this drug has been approved for use in Canada. Other trials indicate that marijuana-derived chemicals may improve MS-related pain, bladder problems, mobility difficulties, and sleeping problems. One small study did not find a therapeutic effect of marijuana extract on MS-related tremor.

Several surveys have been done of marijuana use in people with MS. In these surveys, symptoms that are commonly reported to be improved with smoking marijuana include pain, spasticity, depression, and anxiety. It is important to recognize that surveys such as these are very different from formal clinical studies because people are not evaluated by objective test measures. Rather, people simply give their own assessment; consequently, the results are less reliable than are those obtained in formal clinical trials.

The effects of marijuana on the immune system are not fully understood. Contrary to what might be expected, one study found that marijuana-derived chemicals actually produced immune-stimulating effects. When another study evaluated blood samples from people in the CAMS study, oral THC and marijuana extract did not produce any effects on multiple immune markers

The effects of marijuana-derived chemicals have been investigated in the animal model of MS. In one study, mice with EAE, an experimental form of MS, exhibited spasticity and tremor (3). THC and two other marijuana-derived chemicals reduced both spasticity and tremor in these animals. High doses of marijuana-derived chemicals decreased the overall severity of disease in the MS animal model.

Side Effects

Smoking marijuana has significant adverse effects. Side effects include nausea, vomiting, increased seizure risk, sedation, and poor outcomes with pregnancies. Marijuana smoking may impair driving for up to 8 hours. High doses may decrease reaction time, impair heart function, and cause incoordination and visual difficulties. Chronic marijuana use may impair lung function, cause heart attacks, cause dependence and apathy, and increase the risk of cancer of the lung, head, and neck. Marijuana may increase the sedating effects of medications. It also may increase the activating effect of stimulating medications. *Marijuana use is illegal in many states and countries.*

Conclusion

Studies suggest that marijuana may decrease MS-associated spasticity. It also may be helpful for pain, sleep difficulties, and bladder difficulties. However, marijuana use is associated with significant side effects, and interactions are possible between marijuana and prescription medications. Further studies on the use of marijuana and marijuana-related chemicals in MS are needed. If marijuana is used for MS symptoms, the user should discuss this use with a physician. Users should be aware that marijuana use may be illegal and that prescription medications for MS symptoms may be more effective and safer than marijuana.

Additional Readings

Books

Bowling AC, Stewart TS. *Dietary Supplements and Multiple Sclerosis*. New York: Demos Medical Publishing, 2004, pp. 50–52.
Iversen LL. *The Science of Marijuana*. New York: Oxford University Press, 2000.

Journal Articles

Baker D, Pryce G, Croxford J, et al. Cannabinoids control spasticity and tremor in a multiple sclerosis model. *Nature* 2000;404:84–87.
Baker D, Pryce G, Giovannoni G, et al. The therapeutic potential of cannabis. *Lancet Neurol* 2003;2:291–298.
Bowling AC. Worthless weed or pot of gold? *Int J MS Care* 2004;5:138,166.
Clark AJ, Ware MA, Yazer E, et al. Patterns of cannabis use among patients with multiple sclerosis. *Neurol* 2004;62:2098–2100.
Fox P, Bain PG, Glickman S, et al. The effect of cannabis on tremor in patients with multiple sclerosis. *Neurol* 2004;62:1105–1109.
Katona S, Kaminski E, Sanders H, Zajicek J. Cannabinoid influence on cytokine profile in multiple sclerosis. *Clin Exp Immunol* 2005;140:580–585.
Killestein J, Hoogervorst ELJ, Reif M, et al. Immunomodulatory effects of orally administered cannabinoids in multiple sclerosis. *J Neuroimmunol* 2003; 137:140–143.
Vaney C, Heinzel-Gutenbrunner M, Jobin P, et al. Efficacy, safety and tolerability of an orally administered cannabis extract in the treatment of spasticity in patients with multiple sclerosis: a randomized, double-blind, placebo-controlled, crossover study. *Mult Scler* 2004;10:417–424.
Wade DT, Makela P, Robson P, et al. Do cannabis-based medicinal extracts have general or specific effects on symptoms in multiple sclerosis: a double-blind, randomized, placebo-controlled study on 160 patients. *Mult Scler* 2004; 10:434–441.
Zajicek J, Fox P, Sanders H, et al. Cannabinoids for treatment of spasticity and other symptoms related to multiple sclerosis (CAMS study): multicentre randomised placebo-controlled trial. *Lancet* 2003;362:1517–1526.
Zajicek J, Sanders HP, Wright DE, et al. Cannabinoids in multiple sclerosis (CAMS) study: safety and efficacy data for 12 months follow up. *J Neurol Neursurg Psych* 2005;76:1664–1669.

31

Massage

*M*assage is a healing method that has been used for thousands of years. It was a recommended therapy in ancient China and Egypt. Many common forms of massage now used in the United States are derived from Swedish massage, which was developed by a Swedish physician in the nineteenth century. Massage may be provided on its own, or it may be a component of other forms of alternative healing, including Ayurveda, traditional Chinese medicine, and aromatherapy.

Treatment Method

Massage usually is done on a specially designed table in a warm, quiet room with soft lighting and relaxing music. The individual receiving the massage is partially or completely undressed; a sheet or towel is used to cover parts of the body that are not being massaged. The therapist uses a variety of techniques, including pressing, stroking, rubbing, slapping, and tapping. Oil or lotion usually is used to make the movements smoother.

Massage may be effective through several possible mechanisms. First, massage appears to relax muscles (although only limited studies have formally evaluated this effect). This effect may be helpful for conditions that are worsened by muscle stiffness, such as headaches, neck pain, and low back pain. Also, massage may release chemicals known as *endorphins*, which reduce pain. Through a theoretical process known as *gate control*, which presumes that only a certain number of impulses may reach the brain from a specific body part, stimulation by massage in a painful area may decrease the number of pain impulses received by the brain from that area. Finally, the simple act of touching that occurs with massage may convey positive feelings that are difficult to evaluate rigorously, such as caring, comfort, and acceptance. Touching is a simple and possibly beneficial act that often is missing from interactions between patients and physicians and other mainstream health care providers.

Studies in MS and Other Conditions

Few studies have specifically evaluated massage therapy in people with multiple sclerosis (MS). In a study reported in 1998, 24 people with MS who received massage therapy were compared with those who did not (1). In this small study, massage therapy was associated with multiple benefits, including increased self-esteem, improved social functioning, and reduced anxiety and depression. In addition, those who received massage had better self-perception of their bodies and the progression of their disease. Another small trial found that slow, stroking massage movements over the spine were associated with improvement in anxiety and in the electrophysiologic measures of muscle stiffness (2). A small preliminary study of two people with MS found that massage along with aromatherapy was associated with improvements in mobility, personal hygiene, and dressing ability (3).

Symptoms that may occur with MS have been studied in other conditions. However, nearly all these studies have serious limitations; consequently, the results must not be taken as definitive. Some studies have shown a reduction in stress, anxiety, and depression. It is often stated that spasticity or stiffness in the arms or legs may improve with massage; studies in this area are surprisingly limited. Some studies indicate that abdominal massage may improve constipation. Several forms of pain, including low back pain and cancer-related pain, may improve with massage. The National Cancer Institute recognizes massage as a non-medication therapy for pain.

In addition to its effects on specific symptoms, massage also may have a beneficial effect on self-esteem and overall quality of life through its "healing touch" properties. Dr. Elizabeth Forsythe, an English physician with MS, wrote about her experiences with massage in the book *Multiple Sclerosis: Exploring Sickness and Health*: "Her patience, acceptance, and her remarkable hands began to lessen my loathing for my body. The massage also relieved much of the muscle spasm and tension in my body. Being massaged by somebody known and trusted is a good start to the building or rebuilding of a personal world of trust" (4).

The effects of massage on the immune system are not well understood. Immune stimulation has been reported with massage, but the significance of this effect is not known. In one study, infants with AIDS, an immune-deficiency state, were treated with massage and had a better course than those who did not receive massage.

Side Effects

Massage usually is well tolerated. Minor adverse effects that have been reported include headache, muscle pain, and lethargy. There are also rare, isolated reports of more serious complications, such as bleeding into the liver with deep abdominal massage.

To prevent complications, there are certain conditions for which massage should be avoided or practiced with caution. The following guidelines should be followed:

■ Recent injuries, such as fractures and open skin lesions, should not be massaged.

■ Abdominal massage should be avoided by people with ulcers or enlargement of the liver or spleen.

■ People with fever, infection, clotted blood vessels (thrombosis), and jaundice should avoid massage.

■ Those with cancer, arthritis, and heart disease should consult a physician before receiving massage therapy.

■ Women who are pregnant should only receive massage from therapists who are experienced in pregnancy massage.

Practical Information

Massage often is performed by a therapist, but it also may be done on one's own without a therapist. Massage therapy sessions typically last from 30 to 90 minutes and cost $30 to $60 per hour. The expense of massage therapy is covered by some insurance plans. You can locate a massage therapist in the yellow pages of the telephone book.

More information about massage and qualified massage therapists is available from:

■ The American Massage Therapy Association (www.amtamassage.org), 500 Davis Street, Evanston IL 60201 (877-905-2700)

■ National Certification Board for Therapeutic Massage and Bodywork (www.ncbtmb.com), 1901 South Meyers Road, Suite 240, Oakbrook IL 60181-5243 (800-296-0664)

Conclusion

Massage is a relatively safe, low- to moderate-cost therapy that may have several benefits. Although it has not been extensively studied in MS, limited studies in other conditions suggest that it may be helpful for some MS-associated symptoms, including anxiety, depression, constipation, muscle stiffness (spasticity), low back pain, and other types of pain.

Additional Readings

Books

Ernst E, ed. *The Desktop Guide to Complementary and Alternative Medicine: An Evidence-Based Approach.* Edinburgh: Mosby, 2001.

Oken BS, ed. *Complementary Therapies in Neurology.* London: Parthenon Publishing, 2004.

Vickers A. *Massage and Aromatherapy: A Guide for Health Professionals.* London: Chapman & Hall, 1996.

Weintraub MI, Micozzi MS, eds. *Alternative and Complementary Treatments in Neurologic Illness.* New York: Churchill Livingstone, 2001.

Journal Articles

Brouwer B, de Andrade VS. The effects of slow stroking on spasticity in patients with multiple sclerosis: a pilot study. *Physiother Theory Practice* 1995; 11:13–21.

Hernandez-Reif M, Field T, Field T, et al. Multiple sclerosis patients benefit from massage therapy. *J Bodywork Movement Ther* 1998;2:168–174.

Vanderbilt S. Searching for comfort: alternative therapies and multiple sclerosis. *Massage and Bodywork* 2004;Aug/Sept:50–59.

Walsh E, Wilson C. Complementary therapies in long-stay neurology in-patient settings. *Nursing Standard* 1999;13:32–35.

32

Meditation

$\mathcal{M}$editation is a type of mind–body therapy, a class of therapies that also includes biofeedback, hypnosis, and guided imagery. For thousands of years, meditation has been practiced in some form, especially in the context of religious practice. Also, meditation is one of several components of some complementary and alternative medicine (CAM) therapies, including Ayurveda (which uses transcendental meditation or TM) and traditional Chinese medicine.

Meditation is a way of producing the *relaxation response*, which has been described extensively by Dr. Herbert Benson at the Harvard Medical School and The Mind/Body Medical Institute. The relaxation response is a state of relaxation associated with decreased anxiety, muscle relaxation, and lowering of blood pressure. It is believed to be the opposite of the physiologic response known as the *fight-or-flight response*, characterized by the activation or stimulation of multiple body processes, such as increases in heart rate, blood pressure, and breathing rate.

Treatment Method

Many different meditation methods are used. All these techniques elicit relaxation by focusing concentration, relaxing the body, and diverting attention from stressful thoughts and feelings. One of the simplest strategies is outlined by Dr. Herbert Benson in *The Relaxation Response*:

1. Sit in a comfortable position in a quiet room and close your eyes.
2. Relax your muscles by starting with the feet and slowly working up the body to the face.
3. Each time you exhale, say a word silently.
4. Try to avoid distracting thoughts.
5. Continue this process for 10 to 20 minutes.

Other, more formal, meditation methods include transcendental meditation, mindfulness meditation (or *vipassana*), and meditation techniques associated with Zen (the Chinese word for meditation) and yoga. Mindfulness meditation has been extensively described and researched by Dr. Jon Kabat-Zinn. The relaxation response also may be produced by hypnosis, guided imagery, biofeedback, and prayer, all of which are discussed in detail elsewhere in this book.

Studies in MS and Other Conditions

No studies have formally evaluated the effects of meditation in a large number of people with multiple sclerosis (MS). In one study of 40 people, nine of whom had MS, meditation along with imagery decreased both anxiety and physical complaints during the physical rehabilitation process (1).

Other research studies have examined meditation effects on symptoms that may occur with MS but have involved people with conditions other than MS. It has been found that meditation may improve stress, anxiety, depression, and various types of pain. Although difficult to study formally, feelings of control, empowerment, and self-esteem may develop through meditation. *Progressive muscle relaxation*, a specific process sometimes used in meditation, may improve insomnia.

Interestingly, meditation and other relaxation methods may produce changes in immune function. Various immune-system changes have been described. The precise effects and their impact on MS are not fully understood at this time.

An interesting example of the influence of meditation on immune function was described in a 1985 report (2). A woman experienced in an Eastern religious–type of meditation was given small skin injections of a component of the chickenpox virus. Because she had been exposed to the virus previously, she had, as expected, an immune response to the injection that involved inflammation and redness of skin. Subsequently, she was told to use her meditation skills to attempt to decrease the injection response for a 3-week period. For each week during that time, her skin reaction was reduced, and the activity of her immune cells was decreased.

Meditation has been investigated in a number of other medical conditions. It may improve psoriasis (a skin condition), reduce blood pressure, and improve heart function in people with heart disease. Meditation also has produced some beneficial results in various forms of addiction.

Side Effects

Meditation does not usually involve any serious risks. It may produce difficulties in people with serious psychiatric diseases, such as severe depression and schizophrenia. The state of relaxation elicited by meditation may produce fear of losing control, disturbing thoughts, and anxiety. Meditation should not be used in place of conventional therapy to treat MS or serious MS-associated symptoms.

Practical Information

Meditation may be done independently by following techniques described in books such as *The Relaxation Response*. Classes in meditation techniques often are available through hospitals, health clubs, and community centers. Individual classes are typically 30 to 90 minutes in length and cost $60 to $150 per session. Group sessions are 60 minutes and cost $15 to $35. If meditation is pursued, it is important to keep in mind that it often does not have immediate effects. It may take several weeks or months of practice to achieve significant relaxation.

Conclusion

Meditation is a well-tolerated, low-cost therapy that may provide medical benefits without the use of medication. For people with MS, meditation may be helpful for relieving stress, anxiety, depression, insomnia, and pain. It also may improve self-esteem and feelings of control.

Additional Readings

Books

Benson H. *The Relaxation Response*. New York: HarperTorch, 1976.

Ernst E, ed. *The Desktop Guide to Complementary and Alternative Medicine: An Evidence-Based Approach*. Edinburgh: Mosby, 2001.

Fugh-Berman A. *Alternative Medicine: What Works*. Baltimore: Williams & Wilkins, 1997:167–174.

Kabat-Zinn J. *Wherever You Go, There You Are: Mindfulness Meditation in Everyday Life*. New York: Hyperion, 2005.

Rakel D. Recommending meditation. In: Rakel D, Faass N. *Complementary Medicine in Clinical Practice*. Boston: Jones and Bartlett, 2006.

Weintraub MI, Micozzi MS, eds. *Alternative and Complementary Treatments in Neurologic Illness*. New York: Churchill Livingstone, 2001.

Journal Articles

Mandel Allan R, Keller Sandra M. Stress management in rehabilitation. *Arch Phys Med Rehabil* 1986;67:375–379.

Smith GR, McKenzie JM, Marmer DJ, et al. Psychologic modulation of the human immune response to *Varicella zoster. Arch Int Med* 1985;145:2110–2112.

Zachariae R, Kristensen JS, Hokland P, et al. Effect of psychological intervention in the form of relaxation and guided imagery on cellular immune function in normal healthy subjects: an overview. *Psychother Psychosom* 1990;54:32–39.

33

Music Therapy

*A*s its name implies, music therapy uses music to facilitate healing. This type of therapy has been practiced for thousands of years. It was used in some form in ancient Egypt and ancient Greece. Singing and drumming are also components of shamanic and Native American healing.

In the United States, music therapy degrees were first granted in the 1940s. The National Association for Music Therapy established music therapy as an official discipline in 1950. Conventional medicine has increasingly recognized music therapy. About 5,000 professional and student music therapists practice in the United States.

Treatment Method

In music therapy, people either create or listen to music. The appropriate form of therapy for a specific person is determined by a trained music therapist. Music therapy may be practiced on an individual or group basis. Music is also sometimes used to facilitate imagery (see the chapter "Hypnosis and Guided Imagery").

The mechanism by which music therapy may be therapeutic is not known. Music is known to produce emotional responses. Because the brain pathways for music-associated emotional responses are different from those for verbal communication, music may be a novel way to stimulate emotions, facilitate emotional processing, and produce emotional change. Some of music's benefits may be related to music-induced relaxation. In addition, for people with movement difficulties such as incoordination or walking disorders, music therapy may elicit *entrainment*, which essentially means that moving to the music makes movements more rhythmic, regular, and efficient.

Studies in MS and Other Conditions

Music therapy has undergone limited investigation in multiple sclerosis (MS). One study of 20 people with MS found that music therapy improved self-esteem, depression, and anxiety (1). Another study of 225 people with MS reported that group music therapy may provide psychological support, improve depression and anxiety, and assist in coping with the disease (2). In a small investigational study of people with advanced MS, an indication was noted that music therapy improves respiratory muscle weakness (3).

In people with other conditions, music therapy has produced beneficial effects. Music therapy may have emotional and cognitive benefits. It has been shown to decrease anxiety in some, but not all, studies. Limited studies suggest that music therapy decreases agitation and aggression in people with Alzheimer's disease. Music also may improve cognitive function—it may facilitate learning in children and college students and may improve attention and concentration in people with Alzheimer's disease.

Physical symptoms may benefit from music therapy. Music therapy may be beneficial for walking unsteadiness and incoordination in children and in adults with stroke and Parkinson's disease. In some studies, music therapy has improved several different types of pain.

Several general concepts have emerged from studies of music therapy in medical settings:

- Women's responses may be greater than men's responses.
- Children and adolescents may be more responsive than adults.
- Live music produces a greater effect than does recorded music.
- Music has a greater effect when a limited amount of pain is present.

Side Effects

Music therapy is essentially risk-free, although excessive noise (greater than 90 decibels) may impair hearing and increase blood pressure.

Practical Information

More information about music therapy and qualified music therapists may be obtained from: The American Music Therapy Association (www.music-therapy.org), 8455 Colesville Road, Suite 1000, Silver Spring MD 20910 (301-589-3300).

Conclusion

Music therapy is a safe and inexpensive approach that may be beneficial for some MS symptoms. Although no large definitive studies in people with MS have been undertaken, limited studies in MS and studies in other groups of people suggest that music therapy may be helpful for anxiety, depression, self-esteem, coping, cognitive problems, walking difficulties, incoordination, and pain. Further research of music therapy in MS and other conditions is needed.

Additional Readings

Books

Gaynor ML. *Sounds of Healing: A Physician Reveals The Therapeutic Power of Sounds, Voice, and Music.* New York: Broadway Books, 1999.

Hanser S, Codding P, Eslinger P. Music therapy. In: Weintraub MI, Micozzi MS, eds. *Alternative and Complementary Treatments in Neurologic Illness.* New York: Churchill Livingstone, 2001, pp. 255–267.

Spencer JW, Jacobs JJ. *Complementary and Alternative Medicine: An Evidence-Based Approach.* St. Louis: Mosby, 2003.

Journal Articles

Lengdobler H, Kiessling WR. Group music therapy in multiple sclerosis: initial report of experience. *Psychother Psychosom Med Psychol* 1989;39:369–373 [in German].

Marwick C. Music therapists chime in with data on medical results. *JAMA* 2000;283:731–733.

Schmid W, Aldridge D. Active music therapy in the treatment of multiple sclerosis patients: a matched control study. *J Music Ther* 2004;61:225–240.

Wiens ME, Reimer MA, Guyn HL. Music therapy as a treatment method for improving respiratory muscle strength in patients with advanced multiple sclerosis: a pilot study. *Rehabil Nurs* 1999;24:74–80.

34

Pets

$\mathcal{P}$ets are not necessarily a form of complementary and alternative medicine (CAM). Caring for a pet may be considered a component of one's lifestyle or a hobby. However, caring for a pet may provide health benefits for people with multiple sclerosis (MS) and other medical conditions, even if it usually is not considered in the context of conventional medical care.

Pets are a part of everyday life for many people, but they may provide special benefits for people with medical conditions. The concept that pets may be therapeutic is not new. In the nineteenth century, the nurse Florence Nightingale, who loved pets and had exotic pets of her own, wrote: "A small pet animal is often an excellent companion for the sick ..." (1).

Recently, pets have been used increasingly in medical settings, and studies indicate that they may provide health benefits. The potential therapeutic effects of pets relate to the concepts of *biophilia* and *ecotherapy*. Biophilia is a term that was proposed by Dr. Edward O. Wilson to explain a connection that humans subconsciously need and seek out with other forms of life. According to this concept, human health depends on one's relations with the natural environment. Ecotherapy aims to provide connection, balance, guidance, and healing to people by deepening their relationships with the natural environment.

Pets may improve both physical and emotional disorders. For people with physical disabilities, trained pets, especially dogs, assist by performing physical tasks, such as retrieving items or by stabilizing people who have walking difficulties. Pets are also sometimes used to assist people with physical rehabilitation, which may involve physical, occupational, or speech therapy.

Emotionally, it has been claimed that pets provide "unconditional love"; they are accepting and noncritical companions. Pet ownership has been associated with relaxation. Pets also may improve self-esteem and increase independence, responsibility, and companionship. Pets sometimes are brought into the hospital to provide possible psychological benefits for children.

Studies in MS and Other Conditions

Clinical studies of pets are limited. No large, well-designed studies have been undertaken of pet ownership in people with MS. In other conditions, early studies indicated that pet ownership improved bereavement, lowered the use of medical services, decrease the risk of allergies and asthma in children, decreased the risk of heart disease, and increased survival rates from heart attacks. However, subsequent studies did not support these findings. In children, pet ownership does appear to decrease absenteeism from school.

Side Effects

Pets generally are well tolerated. However, some considerations should be kept in mind. Obviously, people with allergies should avoid pets that provoke allergies, and people who feel uncomfortable or stressed around pets probably would not benefit from their presence. Adequate care and an appropriate amount of space should be provided. Finally, pets should not substitute for the basic emotional needs that should be obtained from humans. They may be used for a certain level of companionship, but this should not lead to social isolation.

Practical Information

More information on pets can be obtained from:

- Canine Companions for Independence (www.caninecompanions.org.), P.O. Box 446, Santa Rosa CA 95402-0446 (800-572-2275)
- Delta Society (www.deltasociety.com), 875 12th Avenue Northeast, Suite 101, Bellevue WA 98055 (425-226-7357)
- Independence Dogs, Inc., 146 State Line Road, Chadds Ford PA 19317 (610-358-2723)

Conclusion

Caring for a pet is a low-risk, low- to moderate-cost activity that may provide some psychological benefits. Trained pets may be helpful to people with weakness, clumsiness, or walking difficulties.

Additional Readings

Journal Articles

Dossey L. The healing power of pets: a look at animal-assisted therapy. *Alt Ther* 1997;3:8–16.

Mayon-White R. Pets—pleasures and problems. *Brit Med J* 2005;331:1254–1255.

McNicholas J, Gilbey A, Rennie A, et al. Pet ownership and human health: a brief review of evidence and issues. *Brit Med J* 2005;331:1252–1254.

Spittler K. A look at "biophilia"—how does nature impact physical and mental health? *Neurol Rev* 2006;Feb:58–59.

35

Pilates Method and the Physicalmind Method

The Pilates method and a variant of Pilates, the Physicalmind method, are two types of bodywork that are intended to increase flexibility and strength. The Pilates method was created during World War I by Joseph H. Pilates, a German inventor, boxer, and dancer. He developed the technique to help soldiers recover from war injuries. In the United States, Pilates has been practiced since the 1920s, and its popularity has grown during the past decade.

In the Pilates method, individuals concentrate on body movements. During exercises, which include more than 500 specific movements, attention is focused on which muscles are used and how they are controlled. An emphasis also is placed on deep, coordinated breathing. The Physicalmind method was developed in response to a lawsuit regarding the Pilates name. In this spin-off of the original technique, more focus is placed on the position of the body. Both the Pilates method and the Physicalmind method require the use of specialized exercise equipment.

Both methods are claimed to have several beneficial effects. They are supposed to improve strength and flexibility without increasing the size of muscles. Consequently, these methods are particularly popular among dancers.

Studies in MS and Other Conditions

No large clinical studies have been undertaken of the Pilates method or the Physicalmind method. Although both methods are used by some people with multiple sclerosis (MS), these techniques have not been specifically investigated in this disease. In one of the few published studies of this therapy, six elite gymnasts at the University of Illinois received 1 month of leap training combined with the Pilates method and pool training (1). This training regimen resulted in an increased height of jumps, improved reaction times, and increased strength. Another small study found improved flexibility after Pilates training (2). Clearly, further studies of the effectiveness of the Pilates method and the Physicalmind method are needed.

Side Effects

It is generally assumed that the Pilates method and the Physicalmind method are well tolerated.

Practical Information

The Pilates method and the Physicalmind method are taught either individually or in small groups. The techniques should be learned from a trained and certified instructor. The exercises may be done individually after receiving training. Adequate training usually requires a total of 20 to 30 sessions; each session generally costs $30 to $70. More information may be obtained from: The Pilates Studio (www.pilates-studio.com), 311 W 43rd Street, Suite 405, New York NY 10036 (800-474-5283).

Conclusion

The Pilates method and the Physicalmind method are low-risk, moderate-cost forms of bodywork. These therapies are claimed to improve strength and flexibility, but few published studies have evaluated their effectiveness.

Additional Readings

Books

Spencer JW, Jacobs JJ. *Complementary and Alternative Medicine: An Evidence-Based Approach*. St. Louis: Mosby, 2003, pp. 196, 580.

Journal Articles

Anonymous. Conditioning by Pilates. *Harvard Women's Health Watch* 1999;6:7.
Hutchinson MR, Tremain L, Christiansen J, et al. Improving leaping ability in elite rhythmic gymnasts. *Med Sci Sports Ex* 1998;30:1543–1547.
Segal NA, Hein J, Basford JR. The effects of Pilates training on flexibility and body composition: an observational study. *Arch Phys Med Rehab* 2004;85:1977–1981.

36

Prayer and Spirituality

Religion has been a fundamental aspect of human culture for tens of thousands of years. Surveys in the United States indicate that nearly 90 percent of the general population believe that there is a God who responds to prayer. Also, nearly 80 percent of the general population and 75 percent of physicians believe that spiritual faith can improve recovery from a disease.

The term *spirituality* refers to devotion to religious values. Prayer is a component of religious practice that may be used to give thanks to or obtain help from a higher power. Prayer is used to attempt to influence processes and events that are beyond human control, including health and disease. Prayer generally is practiced in conjunction with conventional medical care, but followers of some religions, such as the Christian Science Church, pray in lieu of using conventional medicine.

There has been a recent growth in interest about the possible medical relevance of prayer and spirituality. Some of this interest has been due to the research and writings of Dr. Herbert Benson and Dr. Larry Dossey. Important issues that have been raised are whether spirituality improves health and whether prayer can improve the course of a disease or lessen the severity of a specific symptom.

Treatment Method

Most religions involve some type of prayer. Praying may be done individually or in groups. It may be a type of meditation, or may involve recitations of words silently or aloud. One type of prayer that has been studied in medical settings is known as *intercessory prayer*, which involves one person praying for another individual who may be in a different geographic location. It is important to recognize that prayer is one of many components of religious practice and that it may not be effective if done independently of the other aspects of religious belief.

In addition to prayer, spirituality is an active area of research. Whether spiritual belief produces effects beyond those of the placebo response has not been established. It has been claimed that spirituality may be an especially potent means of producing the placebo effect because placebo effects require belief, and religious belief may be the most profound form of belief.

Studies of MS and Other Conditions

The effects of prayer and spirituality on multiple sclerosis (MS) have not been rigorously studied. One frequently described case of MS that appeared to respond dramatically to prayer and faith involved Rita Klaus. Klaus was a nun who was diagnosed with MS in 1960, at the age of 20. Because of the effects of her illness, she was given dispensation of her vows and left the convent. She eventually married and had three children.

Her disease progressed significantly over the years. She wore leg braces, required the use of a wheelchair, and eventually had surgery on her knees to relieve some of the severe stiffness or spasticity in her legs. Her religious faith dwindled with the progression of her disease. She became skeptical of God and religion in general.

At the urging of her husband, she became more committed religiously, prayed regularly, and developed a renewed and more mature faith. Then, one evening in 1986, 26 years after her diagnosis of MS, she prayed for healing of her disease. The following morning, she had unusual warm and itching sensations in her legs. She was able to move her legs and then get out of her wheelchair and walk. The surgical changes in her knees were no longer apparent.

Klaus has not had any recurrent symptoms of MS since that day in 1986. By this account, her MS became inactive, and she also recovered fully from the significant injury to her nervous system that had occurred over the course of 26 years. She returned to her job as a schoolteacher and now gives public lectures on her remarkable experience. Her physician, Dr. Donald Meister, reported that her neurologic examination returned to normal. He is unable to explain her recovery. A urologist found that her urinary system, which had been very abnormal, returned to normal function. The medical documentation of her recovery is reportedly under review by the Vatican.

At the Rocky Mountain Multiple Sclerosis Center, we conducted a survey of spirituality and prayer in more than 1,000 people with MS. The vast majority of the respondents (90 percent) stated that they believed in

God. Within this group, more people (43 percent) believed that God did not play a role in their having MS than believed that God did play a role (28 percent). Of those who believed God played a role in their having MS, a very small percentage (3 percent) thought that MS was a punishment from God. The majority (90 percent) of those who thought that God played a role in their having MS believed that MS was an opportunity from God. Most of the survey respondents (86 percent) stated that they were spiritual. Also, the majority believed in miracles (80 percent) and believed that MS had made them more spiritual (58 percent). In the area of prayer, most of the respondents (87 percent) prayed, and one-half (50 percent) believed that prayer helped control their MS. Areas that were most commonly reported to improve with prayer were anxiety, uncertainty about the disease, and depression. The full results of this survey and a review of the survey results may be viewed on the CAM website of the Rocky Mountain Multiple Sclerosis Center, www.ms-cam.org.

A large, formal clinical study has been conducted in the Midwest to evaluate more fully the subject of prayer in MS. This study of more than 200 people with MS is evaluating the effects of intercessory prayer on physical disability and quality of life. Two groups, are participating in the study, one of which is receiving prayer while the other is not. The results of the study have not yet been published.

Variable results have been obtained in studies of the effects of prayer on other medical conditions. Anxiety and depression, which may occur with MS, may be reduced in those who pray. For anxiety, a therapeutic effect of prayer could be due to the fact that prayer, like meditation, elicits relaxation (see the chapter on "Meditation").

One active area of investigation is the possible influence of intercessory prayer on people with various medical conditions. Interest in this area was stimulated by a widely known study that was conducted in a coronary care unit in San Francisco (1). This 1988 study of nearly 400 people found that those who were prayed for experienced fewer complications, including heart failure, respiratory problems, and use of some types of medication. No effect of prayer was noted on the death rate or the length of hospital stay. This study has been criticized for many reasons, including statistical flaws.

Reviews of the various studies of intercessory prayer have been published (2,3). These reviews conclude that promising results have been obtained, but that the studies have had deficiencies, the results have been variable, and, overall, the results are not definitive. These reviews recommend that further research be conducted in this area through clinical studies using improved methodology.

The effects of spirituality on MS have not been investigated formally. However, religious involvement and spirituality may be beneficial for anxiety and stress, which may occur with MS. In some, but not all studies, religious involvement has been associated with decreased depression. Religious involvement and spirituality also may improve quality of life, decrease the risk of developing some diseases (including high blood pressure and heart disease), decrease mortality rates, and improve coping with or recovery from illness.

Side Effects

Prayer and spirituality generally are safe. Some people have expressed concern that negative thoughts about an individual could lead to negative health outcomes. Prayer and spirituality should not be used in place of conventional medical care.

Conclusion

Prayer and spirituality are low risk and inexpensive. The health effects of these approaches have not been established. Some studies suggest that prayer may be beneficial for anxiety and depression, and that religious involvement and spirituality may decrease anxiety, improve depression, prevent some diseases, decrease mortality rates, improve quality of life, and improve coping with and recovery from illness. A research study has evaluated the effects of intercessory prayer on MS—the results of this study have not yet been published.

Additional Readings

Books

Benson H. *Timeless Healing: The Power and Biology of Belief.* New York: Simon & Schuster, 1996.

Cassileth BR. *The Alternative Medicine Handbook.* New York: W.W. Norton, 1998:292–293, 309–313.

Dossey L. *Reinventing Medicine: Beyond Mind-Body to a New Era of Healing.* San Francisco: HarperCollins, 1999.

Hirshberg C, Barasch MI. *Remarkable Recovery: What Extraordinary Healings Tell Us About Getting Well and Staying Well.* New York: Berkley, 1996.

Kiresuk TJ, Trachtenburg AI, Boucher TA. Psychiatric disorders. In: Oken BS, ed. *Complementary Therapies in Neurology.* London: Parthenon Publishing, 2004, pp. 417–419.

Klaus R. *Rita's Story*. MA: Paraclete Press, 1993.

Mueller P. Religious involvement, spirituality and medicine: subject review and implications for clinical practice. In: Oken BS, ed. *Complementary Therapies in Neurology*. London: Parthenon Publishing, 2004, pp. 189–207.

Spencer JW, Jacobs JJ. *Complementary and Alternative Medicine: An Evidence-Based Approach*. St. Louis: Mosby, 2003.

37

Prokarin

The preparation known as Prokarin was developed by Elaine DeLack, a nurse with multiple sclerosis (MS), who lives in Washington. It is claimed that Prokarin, which was originally named Procarin, improves many MS-related symptoms.

Treatment Method

Prokarin contains histamine and caffeine and is administered by a skin patch applied to the thigh. A patch is used because histamine is not absorbed if it is taken by mouth. In one study, the patch was applied for 8 hours, and two patches were used daily.

Prokarin was developed on the basis of a theory about histamine developed by Dr. Bayard Horton and Dr. Hinton Jonez in the 1940s and 1950s. Histamine treatment presumably decreases allergic reactions and enlarges blood vessels. Caffeine acts as a stimulant.

Studies in MS and Other Conditions

Information about the effectiveness of Prokarin itself is limited. Elaine DeLack claims that her MS was dramatically improved by using Prokarin. Reports have been published of a study of Prokarin in 10 people with MS in Washington State. It is claimed that 8 of the 10 people in this study experienced improvement in MS symptoms that included bladder and bowel difficulties, incoordination, weakness, speech problems, walking unsteadiness, and fatigue.

One published study evaluated the effects of Prokarin use in 55 people with MS (1). It was found that 67 percent of people experienced improvement in MS symptoms after 6 weeks of treatment. Improvement was noted in a wide range of symptoms, including weakness, numbness, walking difficulties, pain, fatigue, and depression. This study is limited by the fact that neither caffeine alone nor a placebo treatment was used. Also, the effectiveness of the therapy was determined by self-assessment, an approach that is subject to inaccuracy.

A placebo-controlled study of Prokarin was reported in 2002 (2). This was a 12-week study of 29 people with MS. Prokarin was reported to improve fatigue. A question raised in the study was whether the fatigue-relieving effect was due to the caffeine in Prokarin. Blood caffeine levels were similar for the Prokarin- and placebo-treated groups. This suggests that caffeine was not the critical factor in decreasing fatigue, but the results of this relatively small study are not conclusive. Prokarin did not produce changes in brain chemistry (as measured by a technique known as MR spectroscopy) and did not improve thinking abilities, walking, or arm coordination.

At the Rocky Mountain Multiple Sclerosis Center, we conducted a web-based survey of Prokarin use among more than 1,300 people with MS. A relatively small fraction of the respondents (125 people, or 9.4 percent), had tried Prokarin. The majority (65 percent) of those who tried Prokarin had subsequently stopped using it. The most common reason (reported by 63 percent) for discontinuing Prokarin was lack of effectiveness. Of those who tried Prokarin, 49 percent reported beneficial effects. The symptoms that were most commonly reported to improve with Prokarin were fatigue, muscle stiffness, urination difficulties, and walking difficulties. The full results of the survey may be viewed on the CAM website of the Rocky Mountain Multiple Sclerosis Center, www.ms-cam.org.

Older reports of histamine treatment for MS, published in the late 1940s and the early 1950s, used intravenous histamine along with another medication (tubocurarine), physical therapy, and allergy testing. Beneficial effects of this multimodality treatment were noted. However, the significance of these findings for histamine treatment alone is not clear because several different therapies were used simultaneously, and strict clinical trial guidelines (such as the use of placebo-treated groups) were not followed.

In response to information about Prokarin's reported benefits, the Clinical Advisory Committee of the Greater Washington Chapter of the National Multiple Sclerosis Society released a statement in 1999. In this statement, physicians and nurses expressed the opinion that they did not believe that Prokarin was beneficial for their MS patients. They also had concerns that Prokarin was being used instead of prescription medications with established effectiveness for treating MS.

Side Effects

Limited information is available on the safety of Prokarin. The histamine in Prokarin may potentially worsen asthma, and there have been reports that Prokarin has caused severe asthmatic attacks. One person taking liore-sal (Baclofen) experienced irritability and loss of appetite while taking Prokarin. Rashes have occurred at the site where the patch is applied.

In the Rocky Mountain Multiple Sclerosis Center survey of Prokarin use, about one-half of respondents (44 percent) noted a rash. Other side effects reported included sleeping difficulties (8 percent), weakness (6 percent), fatigue (6 percent), and walking problems (6 percent). Chest tightness, wheezing, or breathing problems were noted by 1.4 percent. The full results of this survey may be viewed at the CAM website of the Rocky Mountain Multiple Sclerosis Center, www.ms-cam.org.

Prokarin should not be used *instead* of conventional MS medications, especially disease-modifying medications such as glatiramer acetate (Copaxone), interferons (Avonex, Betaseron, Rebif), mitoxantrone (Novantrone), and natalizumab (Tysabri).

Practical Information

Prokarin is available only by prescription and costs between $149 and $249 per month.

Conclusion

Prokarin is expensive, and limited information exists about its safety and effectiveness. One small study suggests that it may improve fatigue. Prokarin should not be used by people with asthma because it contains histamine.

Additional Readings

Journal Articles

Alonso A, Jick SS, Hernan MA. Allergy, histamine 1 receptor blockers, and the risk of multiple sclerosis. *Neurol* 2006;66:572–575.

Gillson G, Richards TL, Wright JV, Smith RB, Wright, JV. A double-blind pilot study of the effect of Prokarin on fatigue in multiple sclerosis. *Mult Scler* 2002;8:30–35.

Gillson G, Wright JV, Ballasiotes G. Transdermal histamine in multiple sclerosis. Part 1: Clinical experience. *Alt Med Rev* 1999;4:424–428.

Horton BT, Wagener HP, Aita JA, et al. Treatment of multiple sclerosis by the intravenous administration of histamine. *JAMA* 1944;124:800–801.

Jonez HD. Management of multiple sclerosis. *Postgrad Med* 1952;2:415–422.

38

Reflexology

Reflexology is a therapy based on applying pressure to specific parts of the foot. It is similar to acupressure and shiatsu. In the United States, reflexology was initially developed in the early 1900s by Dr. William Fitzgerald, an ear, nose, and throat specialist in Connecticut. He named the treatment *zone therapy*. Subsequently, in the 1930s, Eunice Ingham, an American nurse and physical therapist, modified the method and named it *reflexology*. Her nephew, Dwight Byers, is one of the current authorities in this area and is president of the International Institute of Reflexology.

Treatment Method

In reflexology, specific parts of the foot are believed to correspond to different body parts. The application of pressure to reflex points (referred to as *cutaneo-organ reflex points*) on the foot is claimed to affect specific parts of the body. The left foot is associated with the left half of the body, while the right foot is associated with the right half.

Reflexology is intended to improve health by increasing energy flow to specific parts of the body. In this way, it is similar to other healing systems that believe in a life force, such as traditional Chinese medicine and Ayurvedic medicine.

Reflexology usually is provided by a trained reflexologist. It also may be done individually. Sessions usually start with a foot massage and are followed by application of pressure to reflex points.

Studies in MS and Other Conditions

Clinical studies of reflexology are extremely limited. Anecdotal reports exist of people with multiple sclerosis (MS) benefiting from reflexology. One MS clinical study, which was not rigorously conducted, reported the improvement of multiple symptoms through the use of reflexology (1). A larger and more rigorous study, which involved 71 people with MS who were treated for 11 weeks, found improvement in muscle stiffness and sensory and bladder symptoms (2). Limited studies of pain (including headache), anxiety, and premenstrual syndrome have found positive effects, but these studies have serious limitations.

Side Effects

Reflexology is well tolerated, and no serious side effects are known. It should be used with caution by those with foot conditions, including ulcers, gout, arthritis, and vascular disease. Although reflexology usually is not painful, one German study of reflexology use in people after surgery found that the technique occasionally triggered abdominal pain.

Practical Information

Reflexology sessions are 30 to 60 minutes in length. Several informational resources for reflexology exist. Books on the subject are available in bookstores and libraries. Information and lists of trained practitioners are available from: The International Institute of Reflexology, (www.reflexology-use.net), 5650 First Avenue North Street, St. Petersburg FL 33433-2642 (727-343-4811).

Conclusion

Reflexology is a low-risk, low- to moderate-cost therapy. One study in MS found that reflexology improved muscle stiffness and bladder and sensory symptoms. Further studies of reflexology in MS and other conditions are needed.

Additional Readings

Books

Cassileth BR. *The Alternative Medicine Handbook*. New York: W.W. Norton, 1998: 236–239.

Ernst E, ed. *The Desktop Guide to Complementary and Alternative Medicine: An Evidence-Based Approach*. Edinburgh: Mosby, 2001, pp. 66–69.

Spencer JW, Jacobs JJ. *Complementary and Alternative Medicine: An Evidence-Based Approach*. St. Louis: Mosby, 2003, pp. 368, 369, 382, 581.

Vickers A. *Massage and Aromatherapy: A Guide for Health Professionals.* London: Chapman & Hall, 1996.

Journal Articles

Joyce M, Richardson R. Reflexology can help MS. *Int J Alt Compl Med* 1997 July:10–12.

Oleson T, Flocco W. Randomized controlled study of premenstrual symptoms treated with ear, hand, and foot reflexology. *Obstet Gynecol* 1993; 82:906–911.

Siev-Ner I, Gamus D, Lerner-Geva L, et al. Reflexology treatment relieves symptoms of multiple sclerosis: a randomized controlled study. *Mult Scler* 2003; 9:356–361.

39

T'ai Chi

T'ai chi, also known as t'ai chi ch'uan, was developed in China hundreds of years ago and is a component of traditional Chinese medicine. On the surface, t'ai chi appears to be simply slow body movements. In practice, it may provide some of the physical benefits of exercise and the relaxation effects of meditation. T'ai chi has been widely practiced in China for centuries and has recently become popular in the United States.

Treatment Method

T'ai chi may be done individually or in groups. A high level of strength and flexibility are not required because the exercises are based largely on technique. T'ai chi consists of slow, rhythmic body movements. The arms are moved slowly and smoothly in circular movements while weight is shifted from one leg to the other and specific breathing techniques are used. A specified series of movements is known as a *form*. T'ai chi movements are claimed to balance the two opposing forces within the human body, *yin* and *yang*. Performing t'ai chi movements is believed to strengthen and balance the life force, known as *chi* or *qi*.

Studies in MS and Other Conditions

A small 1999 study found that t'ai chi may be beneficial for people with multiple sclerosis (MS) (1). This study, conducted at the American College of Traditional Chinese Medicine in San Francisco, examined the effects of an 8-week t'ai chi group program on 19 people with MS. People were accepted into the study regardless of the severity of their disability. T'ai chi improved emotional and social function and produced physical benefits, with a 21 percent improvement in walking speed and a 28 percent decrease in muscle stiffness. Comments obtained from participants indicated that the group experience itself was an important component of the program. The results of this study are promising, but there are limitations. Specifically, no placebo-treated group was used, and assessment was done by the participants themselves rather than by unbiased observers.

Another MS study evaluated the effects of *mindfulness of movement*, a component of t'ai chi (2). Mindfulness of movement involves developing a moment-to-moment awareness of the quality of breathing, movement, and posture. In the study, eight people with MS were given one-on-one instruction in mindfulness of movement as well as audio and videotape aids. The placebo-treated group, which also included eight people with MS, continued with their current care program. People were assessed before the program and after 3 months. Those who participated in mindfulness of movement showed improvement in multiple symptoms, as assessed by patients and by relatives. Limitations of this study include a relatively large number of people who dropped out of the study, small numbers of people overall in the study, and the lack of objective (blinded) clinicians for assessment. Larger and more rigorous studies of t'ai chi in MS are needed.

The effects of t'ai chi on some MS-related symptoms have been investigated in other conditions. Most of the t'ai chi clinical trials have flaws, thus making it difficult to determine exactly how effective t'ai chi is relative to other forms of exercise. T'ai chi may improve balance and strength and decrease the risk of falls in the elderly. Some of the effects of t'ai chi on walking may be due to increased confidence and decreased fear of falling. Research studies have found that t'ai chi also increases strength and flexibility and may improve heart and lung function. Limited evidence suggests that t'ai chi improves depression, anxiety, and fatigue.

T'ai chi is an interesting example of a therapy that may be clinically effective in spite of the fact that its proposed mechanism of action— balancing and strengthening life energy—is unproven.

Side Effects

T'ai chi does not generally pose any known significant health risk. It could potentially worsen fatigue in people with MS. Also, walking unsteadiness and sensitivity to overheating may require modifications in technique. T'ai chi may strain joints and muscles. T'ai chi should be used with caution or avoided by those with acute low back pain, osteoporosis, significant joint injuries, and bone fractures. One report has been published of a person with MS in whom t'ai chi provoked electrical sensations in the arms and back (known as Lhermitte's sign).

Practical Information

It is easiest to learn t'ai chi through classes. T'ai chi may be practiced by people with significant disabilities, but the pace may need to be slowed. T'ai chi may be practiced individually after the basic techniques have been learned.

T'ai chi classes often are provided through community centers and health clubs. Sessions are typically 60 minutes in length and cost between $15 and $30. Many books on this subject are available.

Conclusion

T'ai chi is a low-risk, low- to moderate-cost therapy. In people with MS, it may increase walking ability, decrease stiffness, and improve social and emotional functioning. Studies in other conditions indicate that t'ai chi increases strength and flexibility, and may improve fatigue, depression, and anxiety. For people with MS who have disabilities that prevent participation in strenuous exercise programs, t'ai chi may be a gentle way to obtain some of the general health benefits of a vigorous workout.

Additional Readings

Books

Cassileth BR. *The Alternative Medicine Handbook*. New York: W.W. Norton, 1998:243–247.

Ernst E, ed. *The Desktop Guide to Complementary and Alternative Medicine: An Evidence-Based Approach*. Edinburgh: Mosby, 2001, pp. 74–76.

Hain TC, Kotsias J, Pai C. T'ai chi: applications to neurology. In: Weintraub MI, Micozzi MS, eds. *Alternative and Complementary Treatments in Neurologic Illness*. New York: Churchill Livingstone, 2001, pp. 248–254.

Spencer JW, Jacobs JJ. *Complementary and Alternative Medicine: An Evidence-Based Approach*. St. Louis: Mosby, 2003.

Journal Articles

Chu DA. Tai chi, qi gong, and reiki. *Phys Med Rehabil Clin N Amer* 2004; 15:773–781.

Husted C, Pham L, Hekking A, et al. Improving quality of life for people with chronic conditions: the example of t'ai chi and multiple sclerosis. *Alt Ther* 1999;5:70–74.

Mills M, Allen J. Mindfulness of movement as a coping strategy in multiple sclerosis. A pilot study. *Gen Hosp Psych* 2000;22:425–431.

40

Therapeutic Touch

Therapeutic touch is an energy-based healing method in which life energy is believed to be manipulated therapeutically by the hands of a practitioner. Delores Krieger, a nurse, and Dora Kunz, a healer and clairvoyant, developed this technique during the 1970s. According to Krieger, therapeutic touch has been taught to more than 40,000 people and is practiced in more than 70 countries.

Therapeutic touch is based on concepts similar to those underlying the religious practice of "laying on of hands," in which healing energy is believed to pass from a healer to another person. Similarly, in therapeutic touch, a practitioner's hands are claimed to evaluate and beneficially alter an individual's energy field. Therapeutic touch is based on a concept of a life force, as are traditional Chinese medicine, Ayurvedic medicine, and some other healing methods. It is a modern variation of some of these ancient healing methods.

Treatment Method

Contrary to its name, therapeutic touch does not actually involve touching. Instead, the practitioners' hands are held 2 to 4 inches from a person's body. Several components make up the therapeutic touch session. After an initial "centering" procedure, in which a practitioner establishes an appropriate state of mind, the therapist's hands are used to evaluate the energy flow. Undesirable energy is subsequently removed by sweeping hand movements, and beneficial energy is transferred from the practitioner to the treated individuals.

Studies in MS and Other Conditions

Many anecdotal reports document the benefits of therapeutic touch. However, limited clinical studies have been undertaken on this technique.

No large clinical studies of therapeutic touch have been conducted in multiple sclerosis (MS). One study of an individual with MS reported improvement in stress and coping after one session of therapeutic touch (1).

Some symptoms that may occur with MS have been evaluated in small studies, reported primarily in nursing journals. Several studies indicate that therapeutic touch may decrease anxiety. Mild beneficial effects in small studies have been reported for pain after surgery, tension headaches, burn-associated pain, and arthritis.

Therapeutic touch has undergone limited investigation in other conditions. One study found that wounds heal more rapidly in those who receive therapeutic touch. Therapeutic touch is endorsed as a comfort-promoting technique by the National League for Nursing. Some of its benefits may be due to the attention and caring of the practitioner. Clearly, more research is needed to determine the effects of therapeutic touch.

The validity of therapeutic touch was questioned in a well-publicized article in the *Journal of the American Medical Association* (JAMA) (2). In this study, a 9-year-old girl, Emily Rosa, along with several other investigators (including her mother and father) evaluated 21 therapeutic touch practitioners. Overall, the practitioners, when blindfolded, were not able to detect when their hands were near the hands of another individual. This study, which has been criticized for having significant methodological flaws, questions the conceptual basis of therapeutic touch.

In another study, it was found that people untrained in therapeutic touch could detect the location of an unseen hand if it was 3 or 4 inches away, but not 6 inches away. Also, at 3 inches, a glass shield led to an inability to detect hand location. The authors concluded that body heat, as opposed to an "energy field," was probably used to determine hand location (3).

Side Effects

No significant adverse effects occur after therapeutic touch. Some practitioners believe that excessive energy may be transferred if a session is too long.

Practical Information

Sessions typically last from 20 to 30 minutes and cost between $30 and $60. Practitioners of therapeutic touch may be found in the phone book under various listings: "therapeutic touch," "health services," "holistic centers," "holistic nurses," and "holistic practitioners." More information about therapeutic touch and practitioners may be obtained from:

■ Nurse Healers Professional Associates Incorporated, P.O. Box 444, Alison Park PA 15101 (412-355-8476)
■ American Massage Therapy Association (www.massagetherapy.org), 500 Davis Street, Evanston IL 60201 (877-905-2700)

Conclusion

Therapeutic touch is a low-risk, low- to moderate-expense technique. It has not undergone formal clinical trial testing in MS. Suggestive beneficial effects have been reported for anxiety and pain, but further research is needed to determine the effectiveness of this therapy.

Additional Readings

Books

Ernst E, ed. *The Desktop Guide to Complementary and Alternative Medicine: An Evidence-Based Approach.* Edinburgh: Mosby, 2001.
Leskowitz E. Therapeutic touch in neurology. In: Weintraub MI, Micozzi MS, eds. *Alternative and Complementary Treatments In Neurologic Illness.* New York: Churchill Livingstone, 2001, pp. 234–240.
Spencer JW, Jacobs JJ. *Complementary and Alternative Medicine: An Evidence-Based Approach.* St. Louis: Mosby, 2003.

Journal Articles

Krieger D. Healing with therapeutic touch. *Alt Ther* 1998;4:87–92.
Long R, Bernhardt P, Evans W. Perception of conventional sensory cues as an alternative to the postulated 'human energy field' of therapeutic touch. *Sci Rev Alt Med* 1999;3:53–61.
Payne MB. The use of therapeutic touch with rehabilitation clients. *Rehabil Nursing* 1989;14:69–72.
Rosa L, Rosa E, Sarner L, et al. A close look at therapeutic touch. *JAMA* 1998; 279:1005–1010.

41

Toxins

Over the years, it has been proposed that many toxins may cause multiple sclerosis (MS) or worsen its symptoms. Recent reports have associated MS with aspartame use and mercury from dental amalgam, both of which are discussed elsewhere in this book. It also has been claimed that MS is provoked by cosmetics or by chemicals in the environment in the form of pollution, aerosol sprays, low levels of formaldehyde, and fumes from solvents. In food, it has been claimed that additives and low levels of residual fertilizers and pesticides may be important. On the basis of concerns about toxic causes for MS and other diseases, an entire field known as *clinical ecology* has emerged.

Treatment Method

Many approaches have been proposed to decrease exposure to specific toxins or to decrease levels of toxins in the body. Avoiding aspartame in the diet and removing dental amalgam are sometimes recommended for people with MS. Other approaches claimed to be beneficial for MS include detoxifying therapies such as chelation therapy and colon therapy, also discussed elsewhere in this book, and the avoidance of processed foods, tap water, aerosol sprays, potent housecleaning products, synthetic fabrics, and gas appliances.

Studies in MS and Other Conditions

There is no strong scientific or clinical evidence that specific toxins or exposures—including organic solvents, other chemical compounds, welding, or exposure to electromagnetic fields—play an important role in causing MS or worsening its symptoms. The possible role of zinc or other metals in MS was raised by a study of workers at a manufacturing plant who were exposed to zinc and developed MS. Subsequent studies have not shown a definite association of MS with zinc or other metals. Similarly, no well-documented links exist between MS and aspartame or mercury (see the chapters on these topics).

When considering possible toxins and toxic injury to the body, it is important to recognize that the body has powerful tools to defend itself against toxins. The liver has biochemical mechanisms for converting toxic chemicals to nontoxic chemicals, and the kidneys are able to remove potential toxins from the body by excreting them in the urine. In addition, all cells in the body, including nerve cells, are very resilient and have mechanisms for combating toxins. Consequently, the chances of exposure to chemicals that can cause significant nervous system injury is believed to be extremely low, especially in developed countries.

Conclusion

No toxins have been identified that cause MS or provoke MS symptoms. Although a variety of techniques have been proposed to decrease toxin levels or to decrease exposure to toxins, no studies demonstrate that these techniques produce clinical benefits for people with MS.

Additional Readings

Books

Pryse-Phillips W, Costello F. The epidemiology of multiple sclerosis. In: Cook SD, ed. *Handbook of Multiple Sclerosis*. New York: Marcel Dekker, 2001, pp. 15–31.

Journal Articles

Schaumburg HH, Spencer PS. Recognizing neurotoxic disease. *Neurology* 1987; 37:276–278.

42

Tragerwork

Tragerwork is a form of bodywork. It is also known as Trager, the Trager approach, and Trager psychophysical integration. The technique was developed by Dr. Milton Trager, a physician as well as a boxer, acrobat, dancer, and follower of Maharishi Mahesh Yogi (see the chapter on "Ayurveda"). Tragerwork sometimes is recommended specifically for people with MS and other neurological disorders.

Treatment Method

Tragerwork is designed to change body habits that limit movement or produce muscle pain. Using this treatment, an individual lies on a table while a therapist uses light massage in combination with shaking, bouncing, and rocking movements of the body. This process is believed to produce relaxation and allow one to move with less effort and more grace. Tragerwork therapists also provide instruction in "Mentastics" (a shortened version of "mental gymnastics"), a regimen of self-directed movements that maintain the feelings developed in the treatment sessions. Tragerwork attempts to increase freedom of movement through these methods.

Studies in MS and Other Conditions

Although Tragerwork sometimes is recommended for people with multiple sclerosis (MS), it has not been specifically investigated in this area. There are anecdotal reports of benefit in people with MS, but few published studies have evaluated the effects of Tragerwork on any medical condition. One study found that people with lung disease had improvement in some measures of lung function after Tragerwork (1). The significance of this finding is not clear because the study was small and did not include a placebo-treated control group. In another preliminary study of headache, which did include a control group, Trager treatment was associated with decreased headache frequency, improvement in the quality of life, and decreased use of headache medication (2). In a study of people with spinal cord injury and shoulder pain from wheelchair use, shoulder pain was decreased with either acupuncture or Tragerwork (3).

Side Effects

Limited clinical studies have evaluated the effects of this therapy. Generally it appears to be well tolerated, but people with MS may experience dizziness and nausea with the rocking movements.

Practical Information

Sessions typically last 60 to 90 minutes and cost between $50 and $70. A series of treatment sessions often is recommended. More information about Tragerwork may be obtained from:

- The Trager Institute (www.trager.com), 21 Locust Avenue, Mill Valley CA 94941 (415-388-2688)
- Trager International (www.trager.com), 24800 Chagrin Blvd., Suite 205, Beachwood OH 44122 (216-896-9383)

Conclusion

Tragerwork is a low-risk, moderate-cost form of bodywork. Although there are anecdotal reports of beneficial effects from this therapy, it has not been formally studied in MS. Preliminary studies indicate that it may improve headaches, decrease shoulder pain, and improve lung function.

Additional Readings

Journal Article

Dyson-Hudson TA. Acupuncture and Trager psychophysical integration in the treatment of wheelchair user's shoulder pain in individuals with spinal cord injury. *Arch Phys Med Rehabil* 2001;82:1038.

Foster KA, Liskin J, Cen S, et al. The Trager approach in the treatment of chronic headache: a pilot study. *Alt Ther Health Med* 2004;10:40–46.

Juhan D. Multiple sclerosis: The Trager approach. *Trager Newsletter.* February 1993;1–7.

Witt PL, MacKinnon J. Trager psychophysical integration. A method to improve chest mobility of patients with chronic lung disease. *Phys Ther* 1986; 66:214–217.

43

Vitamins, Minerals, and Other Nonherbal Supplements

The use of vitamins, minerals, and other supplements is both popular and controversial. Surveys of people with multiple sclerosis (MS) indicate that the use of supplements is one of the most common forms of complementary and alternative medicine (CAM). Much of their popularity probably is due to their accessibility. Supplements are easily purchased from grocery stores, health food stores, and drug stores, and using supplements does not require seeing a practitioner.

The potential benefits of supplements are frequently exaggerated by vendors and other proponents of supplements, and the possible uses of supplements in MS are sometimes based on incorrect information about the disease process. In conventional medicine, supplements have been viewed typically with skepticism. Supplements are now undergoing more serious investigation, and supplements are now recommended for preventing or treating a limited number of conditions on the basis of recent research studies.

Background Information

Vitamins are chemicals that are used for many of the body's fundamental chemical processes. In spite of the fact that they are present in only very small quantities, vitamins are absolutely necessary for normal body function. Thirteen vitamins are "essential," which means that the body does not have the biochemical machinery to synthesize them; these vitamins must therefore be consumed in the diet. Most vitamins come from animal or plant foods. The 13 essential vitamins are the eight B vitamins and vitamins A, C, D, E, and K. Most vitamins are water-soluble. The four fat-soluble vitamins are A, D, E, and K.

212

Minerals are also important for maintaining the body's fundamental chemical processes. Minerals originate in soil and water and are incorporated into plants and animals. The minerals needed in large quantities—known as "major minerals"—include calcium, chloride, magnesium, phosphorus, potassium, sodium, and sulfur. Those required in small quantities—the "trace elements"—include chromium, fluoride, iron, selenium, and zinc. A total of 18 trace elements are considered essential.

In addition to vitamins and minerals, other types of supplements are available. Herbs are an especially popular supplement. Other categories of supplements include hormones, antioxidants, amino acids, and enzymes.

How Much Is Needed?

Much of the controversy in the supplement field centers around how much of a particular vitamin or mineral should be consumed daily. The Food and Nutrition Board of the National Academy of Sciences determines the Recommended Daily Allowances (RDAs), Adequate Intakes (AIs), or other similar values for vitamins and minerals (Table 43.1). These values, which have been revised recently, are the daily intake needed to prevent deficiency and possibly provide health benefits.

Some proponents of supplements claim that the RDAs are too low and that higher daily doses are needed. These higher doses of vitamins and minerals are known as *megadoses*. In general, no strong evidence supports megadoses. Importantly, high doses of some vitamins and minerals may produce adverse effects (Table 43.2).

Are Adequate Amounts of Vitamins and Minerals Available in Food?

For a healthy adult, a well-balanced diet should be adequate because it contains enough vitamins and minerals to meet the RDA. It is not clear that supplements are necessary in this situation. However, supplementation may play an important role in other circumstances. For example, if the diet is not well balanced or is low in quantity, the RDA may not be met, and supplementation is important. Also, people with certain conditions may benefit from vitamin or mineral doses that are higher than the RDA; these people may not consume these doses in spite of a well-balanced diet. Examples of this situation are folic acid supplements for pregnant women and vitamin D and vitamin B_{12} supplements for the elderly.

TABLE 43.1. *Recommended Daily Allowance (RDA), Adequate Intake (AI), and Tolerable Upper Intake Levels (ULs) for Adults*

	RDA/AI				
	Men	**Women**	**Pregnant**	**Lactating**	**UL**
VITAMINS					
Biotin					
(Vitamin H)	30 mcg	30 mcg	30 mcg	35 mcg	ND
Choline	550 mg	425 mg	450 mg	550 mg	3.5 g
Cobalamin					
(Vitamin B$_{12}$)	2.4 mcg	2.4 mcg	2.6 mcg	2.8 mcg	ND
Folate					
(Vitamin B$_9$)	400 mcg	400 mcg	600 mcg	500 mcg	1,000 mcg
Niacin					
(Vitamin B$_3$)	16 mg	14 mg	18 mg	17 mg	35 mg
Pantothenic acid					
(Vitamin B$_5$)	5 mg	5 mg	6 mg	7 mg	ND
Pyridoxine	1.2–1.3 mg	1.3–1.5 mg	1.9 mg	2.9 mg	100 mg
(Vitamin B$_6$)					
Riboflavin	1.3 mg	1.1 mg	1.4 mg	1.6 mg	ND
(Vitamin B$_2$)					
Thiamine	1.2 mg	1.1 mg	1.4 mg	1.4 mg	ND
(Vitamin B$_1$)					
Vitamin A	~3,000IU	~2,300 IU	~2,500 IU	~4,300 IU	~10,000 IU
	(900 mcg)	(700 mcg)	(770 mcg)	(1,300 mcg)	(3,000 mcg)
Vitamin C	90 mg	75 mg	85 mg	120 mg	2,000 mg
Vitamin D	200–600 IU	200–600 IU	200 IU	200 IU	2,000 IU
	(5–15 mcg)	(5–15 mcg)	(5 mcg)	(5 mcg)	(50 mcg)
Vitamin E	22 IU	22 IU	22 IU	28 IU	1,500 IU
	(15 mg)	(15 mg)	(15 mg)	(19 mg)	(1,000 mg)
Vitamin K	120 mcg	90 mcg	90 mcg	90 mcg	ND
MINERALS					
Calcium	1,000–1,200 mg	1,000–1,200 mg	1,000 mg	1,000 mg	2,500 mg
Chromium	30–35 mcg	20–25 mcg	30 mcg	45 mcg	ND
Copper	900 mcg	900 mcg	1,000 mcg	1,300 mcg	10,000 mcg
Fluoride	4 mg	3 mg	3 mg	3 mg	10 mg
Iodine	150 mcg	150 mcg	220 mcg	290 mcg	1,100 mcg
Iron	8 mg	8–18 mg	27 mg	9 mg	45 mg
Magnesium	400–420 mg	310–320 mg	350–360 mg	310–320 mg	350 mg
Manganese	2.3 mg	1.8 mg	2.0 mg	2.6 mg	11 mg
Molybdenum	45 mcg	45 mcg	50 mcg	50 mcg	2,000 mcg
Phosphorous	700 mg	700 mg	700 mg	700 mg	3–4 g
Selenium	55 mcg	55 mcg	60 mcg	70 mcg	400 mcg
Zinc	11 mg	8 mg	11 mg	12 mg	40 mg

IU, international units; mcg, micrograms; mg, milligrams; g, grams; ND, not able to determine due to lack of information about adverse effects.

TABLE 43.2   *Doses of Vitamins and Minerals to Avoid*

Vitamins and Minerals	Doses to Avoid
Vitamin A (beta-carotene)	Greater than 10,000 IU/day may produce multiple toxic effects, especially in pregnant women (birth defects)
Vitamin B_3 (niacin)	Greater than 35 mg/day may produce nausea, flushing, and other toxic effects
Vitamin B_6 (pyridoxine)	Greater than 50 mg/day may produce nerve injury
Vitamin C	Greater than 2,500 mg/day may produce diarrhea and kidney stones
Vitamin D	Greater than 2,000 IU/day may produce kidney injury, excessive blood levels of calcium, and other toxic effects
Vitamin E	Greater than 1,000 mg (1,500 IU)/day may produce bleeding complications, upset stomach, and fatigue
Selenium	Greater than 400 mcg/day may produce multiple toxic effects

Vitamins and Minerals Interact with Each Other

Vitamin and mineral supplements have several other significant features that must be taken into account. First, complex interactions occur between vitamins and minerals. As a result, high doses of a single vitamin or mineral may be harmful or ineffective. For example, excessive vitamin C intake may affect the body's ability to absorb copper, and high doses of vitamin B_1 may produce deficiencies of vitamins B_2 and B_6. Also, calcium cannot be utilized for bone health without adequate levels of vitamin D.

Supplements and MS

Supplements are one of the most popular forms of CAM used by people with MS. The largest and most detailed survey of dietary supplement use among people with MS was conducted at the Rocky Mountain Multiple Sclerosis Center. Of the respondents to this survey, more than 90 percent had used dietary supplements since being diagnosed with MS, and more than 80 percent were using some type of dietary supplement at the time of the survey. The full results of the survey are available at www.ms-cam.org, the CAM website of the Rocky Mountain Multiple Sclerosis Center.

Several errors are frequently made in recommending supplements for use in MS. First, recommendations are sometimes haphazard and random; little or no justification is given for a long (and expensive!) list of supplements. When a justification is given, it is sometimes stated that MS is an immune disease and that immune-stimulating supplements are therefore needed. In fact, MS is an immune disease, but it is characterized by too *much*, not too little, immune activity. As a result, immune-stimulating supplements actually may be harmful for MS. Similarly, supplements that may affect the immune system are sometimes recommended for MS as well as cancer and AIDS. Once again, all three diseases do involve the immune system, but people with cancer and AIDS may benefit from *stimulation* of the immune system, whereas people with MS may benefit from its *suppression*.

It is sometimes mistakenly assumed that if a deficiency of a vitamin or mineral impairs the function of the immune system or nervous system, an excess of that same vitamin or mineral will be beneficial to the immune system or nervous system and thus will be therapeutic for MS. In other words, it is assumed that if a little is good, a lot is better. In fact, high doses of vitamins and minerals probably have very limited uses.

A good example of this dosing issue as it relates to the nervous system is that of vitamin B_6 (pyridoxine). A deficiency of vitamin B_6 impairs nervous-system function. However, an excess of vitamin B_6 also *injures* the nervous system and may actually produce symptoms similar to those of MS. Thus, for vitamin B_6 and the nervous system, a normal level is desirable, and either a deficiency or an excess may be harmful.

In the case of immune-system function, seemingly paradoxical situations may arise with regard to supplement doses. For example, vitamin B_7 (biotin) is important for maintaining a healthy immune system; however, a *deficiency* of vitamin B_7 appears to be *beneficial* for animals with EAE, an experimental form of MS. On the other hand, supplementation with either selenium or zinc, two minerals also involved in immune-system function, may worsen EAE. On the basis of this limited scientific information, it could be argued that a state of deficiency of immune-relevant vitamins and minerals may be beneficial for MS, and a state of excess of these nutrients may be harmful. In fact, in one study, malnutrition was found to be a highly effective therapy for the animal model of MS. This information is not provided as a recommendation for people with MS to malnourish themselves or induce deficiency states for particular nutrients! Rather, it is provided to illustrate the complexities of vitamin and mineral dosing for specific diseases such as MS.

Vitamin and mineral supplements are clearly necessary for people with MS who have an inadequate diet. This may occur for a variety of reasons, and may be particularly prevalent in those with more severe disability. With a poor diet, supplementation is essential to ensure an adequate intake of essential nutrients.

The most conservative approach to supplement use in MS is to avoid all supplements (except in people who clearly are nutritionally deficient). The rationale behind this view is that the effectiveness and safety of supplements has not been fully investigated in MS. Thus, according to this view, supplements should not be used, because they may be of no benefit and may actually be harmful.

Principles of Supplement Use in MS

Several steps should be taken when considering supplement use. Objective information should be obtained about the components of the supplement and the claimed health benefits. It must be recognized that, in spite of some claims, no supplement has been fully investigated as benefiting MS. In addition, the use of supplements should be discussed with a physician.

Vitamins

Antioxidant Vitamins Generally (Vitamins A, C, and E)

Relevance to MS.   Among all categories of dietary supplements, antioxidant vitamins were among those used most frequently by a large group of people with MS who were surveyed through a study at the Rocky Mountain Multiple Sclerosis Center (the full results of this survey may be seen at www.ms-cam.org). Antioxidant vitamins include:

- Vitamin A or beta-carotene (a chemical converted to vitamin A)
- Vitamin C
- Vitamin E

These vitamins act on *free radicals*, chemicals that can damage cells in the brain and other organs of the body. For years, it has been proposed that free radicals may play an important role in aging, aging-related diseases, and many other conditions, including MS.

Antioxidants have various actions on the immune system and nervous system—some of these effects could be beneficial for people with MS. Specifically, free radicals may play an important role in MS—using antioxidants to decrease the harmful effects of free radicals may be beneficial. In MS, one type of immune cell, the macrophage, injures the myelin coating on nerve cells by releasing free radicals. Also, the axon—the central part of the nerve cell—is injured in MS, and free radicals may be important in causing axonal injury. In addition, immune cells are activated by the chemical products of free-radical injury to the walls (or membranes) of cells. In the animal model of MS, EAE, growing evidence suggests that free radicals are involved, and that some antioxidant compounds decrease the severity of EAE. Biochemical studies indicate that free-radical damage occurs in people with MS. Thus, multiple scientific and clinical studies indicate that antioxidants may be beneficial to the MS disease process.

Theoretical reasons exist why antioxidants could be *harmful* for MS. Several antioxidants stimulate components of the immune system, including cells known as *macrophages* and *T cells*. These cells are already too active in MS—further activation could, in theory, worsen the disease or antagonize the effects of MS medications such as glatiramer acetate (Copaxone), interferons (Avonex, Betaseron, Rebif), mitoxantrone (Novantrone), or natalizumab (Tysabri).

Although recent basic science and animal-model studies in the area of antioxidants and MS have produced encouraging results, no rigorous clinical trial of antioxidants in MS has yet been undertaken. Limited research results are sometimes used as evidence for the safety of antioxidants in MS. One study found that antioxidant use (vitamin C, vitamin E, and selenium) for 5 weeks in 18 people with MS was *not* associated with worsening of the disease (1). However, this was only a single, short-term study of a relatively small number of people. Another argument for antioxidant safety in MS is that EAE, an animal model of MS, appears to be improved with some types of antioxidant therapy. The animal model of MS is not a perfect model—thus, encouraging results of experimental therapies in this model must be tested in the actual human disease before these therapies are broadly recommended for people with MS. To improve our understanding in this area, multiple trials of antioxidants in MS are underway or are being planned.

With the limited information available at this time, it is reasonable for people with MS to consume antioxidants with care. For people with MS, one reasonable approach is to *not* take antioxidant supplements, but rather to obtain antioxidants through food, specifically fruits and vegetables. Individualized information about fruit and vegetable intake may be obtained at www.mypyramid.gov (see the chapter on "Diets and Fatty Acid Supplements"). General daily recommendations are two to four servings of fruits and three to five servings of vegetables. This dietary intake may result in adequate, but not excessive, levels of antioxidants, and may provide other health benefits.

If people with MS choose to use antioxidant vitamin supplements, it is reasonable to take modest doses. Modest daily doses of these vitamins are:

- Vitamin A—5,000 IU or less
- Vitamin C—90 to 120 milligrams or less
- Vitamin E—100 IU or less

(For vitamin E, conversions may be made between the different forms and units. For lower, nontoxic doses, 1 milligram of alpha-tocopherol = 1.5 IU of natural vitamin E = 2.2 IU of synthetic vitamin E. For higher and potentially toxic doses, 1 milligram of alpha-tocopherol = 1.1 IU of synthetic vitamin E = 1.5 IU of natural vitamin E.)

High daily doses of certain antioxidants should definitely be avoided because of possible toxic side effects (see Table 43.2):

- Greater than 10,000 IU of vitamin A may produce multiple toxic effects, including headache, blurred vision, nausea, and liver injury.
- Greater than 10,000 IU of vitamin A in pregnant women may produce birth defects.
- Greater than 2,500 milligrams of vitamin C may cause diarrhea, abdominal bloating, and kidney stones.
- Greater than 1,000 mg (1,500 IU) of vitamin E may produce stomach upset, bleeding problems, and other difficulties

Other important precautions about antioxidant vitamin use should be noted. Vitamin A or beta-carotene supplements should be avoided or used cautiously by smokers because two studies indicate that beta-carotene supplements increase the risk of death and lung cancer in smokers. Vitamin E may inhibit blood clotting and thus should be avoided by people with bleeding disorders, people taking blood-thinning medications (such as warfarin or Coumadin), and people undergoing surgery. Vitamin C may decrease the effectiveness of blood-thinning medications.

As noted, clinical trials of antioxidants in MS are underway or are being planned. The results from such studies will have important practical applications. If antioxidant supplements are found to be beneficial, they could be recommended; if they are found to be harmful, their use could be discouraged; if they have no effect, they could be avoided and money could be saved or spent on some other type of treatment.

Vitamin E and Polyunsaturated Fatty Acids

It is sometimes recommended that people with MS increase their intake of polyunsaturated fatty acids, as discussed in the "Diet and Fatty Acid Supplements" chapter. Polyunsaturated fatty acid intake may be increased by modifying the diet or by taking fatty acid supplements, such as evening primrose oil, sunflower oil, or fish oil. A potential problem with polyunsaturated fatty acids is that they increase the need for vitamin E. As a result, if polyunsaturated fatty acids are a large part of the diet, or if fatty acid supplements are taken, supplementation with a relatively small amount of vitamin E may be necessary. It is recommended that 0.6 to 0.9 IU of vitamin E should be taken for every gram of polyunsaturated fatty acids consumed. Therefore, if one consumes 25 grams of polyunsaturated fatty acids daily, 15 to 22 IU of vitamin E are needed daily. It is sometimes recommended that people take very high vitamin E doses (2,000 IU or higher) if they are supplementing with polyunsaturated fatty acids—as can be seen from these calculations, such high doses are not needed. For most people who are enriching their diet with polyunsaturated fatty acids, 100 IU of vitamin E should be more than adequate to protect against vitamin E deficiency.

Vitamin E is present in some polyunsaturated fatty acid preparations, including evening primrose oil. The label on the bottle of evening primrose oil should indicate the content of vitamin E.

Vitamin C

The Common Cold.   It is sometimes claimed that vitamin C prevents or decreases the severity of the common cold. This is potentially important to people with MS, because viral infections may trigger MS attacks. However, the effects of vitamin C on the common cold are unclear. Also, because vitamin C stimulates the immune system, high doses of vitamin C supplements are theoretically risky for people with MS. Because of its unclear effects on treating the common cold, and its theoretical risks for worsening MS, it is reasonable for people with MS to be cautious about vitamin C use. If vitamin C is used, orange juice (50 milligrams of vitamin C per half cup of orange juice) or supplements in low doses (90 to 120 milligrams or less daily) may be reasonable.

Urinary Tract Infections.   Vitamin C supplements are sometimes recommended for preventing or treating urinary tract infections (UTIs), which occur frequently in some women with MS. This recommendation is based on the idea that vitamin C, also known as ascorbic acid, makes the urine acidic and thus inhospitable for bacteria. However, there is no definitive evidence that the use of vitamin C supplements produces acidic urine or decreases the chance of developing a UTI.

More evidence exists for cranberry juice (see the chapter on "Herbs") than for vitamin C in preventing UTIs. If an actual infection is present, prescription antibiotics should definitely be used, because people with MS may have serious complications from UTIs.

Vitamin D and Calcium

Vitamin D supplements may be underutilized by people with MS. Vitamin D has two important properties that are relevant to MS. First, it is involved in maintaining bone density, and people with MS are at risk for decreased bone density. Also, vitamin D acts to suppress the immune system and may therefore have a beneficial effect on the disease process.

Vitamin D is considered a hormone as well as a vitamin. A crucial step in the formation of vitamin D is sun exposure. In the skin, the energy of sunlight is used in a chemical reaction that produces the active form of vitamin D. Consequently, sunlight is necessary for adequate vitamin D production, and inadequate sunlight may lead to vitamin D deficiency. Only 10 to 15 minutes of casual sunlight exposure daily is needed.

Vitamin D is well recognized for its role in maintaining the health of bones. Vitamin D and calcium work together to make dense, strong bones. Low levels of vitamin D may lead to severely decreased bone density, a condition known as *osteoporosis*. A less severe form of decreased bone density is referred to as *osteopenia*.

Although studies of osteoporosis often focus on elderly women, it is increasingly recognized that osteoporosis affects many other population groups. Among people with MS, several possible risk factors exist for osteoporosis and low vitamin D levels:

■ People with MS are more likely to be women and to be less physically active than the general population; women and inactive people are at increased risk for osteoporosis.

■ It has been reported that vitamin D intake is inadequate in 80 percent of people with MS, and that blood levels of vitamin D are low in people with MS.

■ Forty percent of people with MS have no sunlight exposure in an average week.

■ Steroids, which are sometimes used to treat MS attacks, may cause osteoporosis. The significance of this steroid effect is unclear in people with MS.

Given these multiple factors, one would expect an increased prevalence of osteoporosis in people with MS. In fact, this has been found in several studies. Bone density is decreased in people with MS, and the loss of bone density over time is greater in people with MS than in the general population. Based on bone density measurements, an estimated two- to threefold increased risk of fractures exists in people with MS. An increased risk of bone fractures with no known trauma also exists in MS. These types of fractures are indicators of decreased bone density.

In addition to its effects on bone, vitamin D may have an important influence on the immune system. A possible association between MS and vitamin D deficiency has been proposed since the early 1970s. Because vitamin D suppresses the immune system, it may be beneficial for MS and other autoimmune diseases in which the immune system is excessively active. In EAE, an animal model of MS, vitamin D supplementation prevents and slows the progression of the disease, whereas vitamin D deficiency worsens the disease. In studies of large groups of people (known as *epidemiologic studies*), increased sunlight exposure has been associated with decreased risk of developing MS or dying from MS. Epidemiologic studies also have shown that the risk of developing MS is lower in women who take vitamin D supplements than in those who do not use vitamin D supplements. Interestingly, animal models of two other autoimmune diseases, diabetes and lupus, also are improved by vitamin D supplementation.

Limited human studies have been undertaken of the effect of vitamin D on MS. One older study evaluated the effect of vitamin D supplementation on the frequency of attacks in 10 people with MS (2). Vitamin D treatment decreased the rate of attacks. It is not possible to draw firm conclusions from this study because it did not include a placebo-treated group, and the treatment also involved cod-liver oil, which contains omega-three fatty acids that may be beneficial for MS, as discussed in the chapter on diet. A preliminary study of 11 people with MS found that 6 months of treatment with a form of vitamin D (19-nor) did not produce clear clinical benefits and did not significantly decrease disease activity observed by magnetic resonance imaging (MRI) scanning (3). A small study of *calcitriol*, which is the active form of vitamin D, reported that this compound was generally safe and well tolerated in people with MS for up to 1 year (4). This study was not designed to determine if calcitriol had therapeutic effects in MS. Large, rigorously designed studies of vitamin D therapy in MS are needed.

Several geographic studies indicate a possible association of vitamin D with MS. It is well known that the prevalence of MS generally increases with an increased distance from the equator. Many hypotheses have been proposed to explain this observation. One is that, as the distance from the equator increases, the sunlight exposure, and therefore the average level of vitamin D, decreases.

Some studies indicate decreased MS prevalence with increased sunlight exposure. In Switzerland, MS is less common at high altitudes than at low altitudes. More ultraviolet light exposure occurs at high altitudes, and perhaps this increases vitamin D levels and thereby decreases the risk of MS. MS is relatively common in Norway except among people who live on the Atlantic coast. People on the coast are more likely to eat fish, which contain relatively high levels of vitamin D. Thus, dietary vitamin D may decrease the risk of developing MS among the coastal people.

These effects also could be due to omega-three fatty acids in fish (see the chapter on "Diet and Fatty Acid Supplements").

If decreased bone density or decreased vitamin D intake is a concern, it should be discussed with a physician. Bone density may be measured by special diagnostic tests, one of which is known as *bone densitometry*.

Supplements of vitamin D usually are taken with calcium. The Adequate Intake (AI) of vitamin D is 200 to 600 IU daily; that of calcium is 1,000 to 1,200 milligrams daily. If vitamin D and calcium supplements are taken, the doses should be discussed with a physician or other health care provider. Prescription medications and, in postmenopausal women, hormone replacement therapy may be indicated. High doses of vitamin D should be avoided because they may cause fatigue, abdominal cramps, nausea, vomiting, kidney damage, high blood pressure, and multiple other toxic effects. Also, calcium and iron should not be taken together because these minerals may interfere with each other's absorption.

Vitamin B_{12}

For years, it has been proposed that vitamin B_{12} deficiency plays a role in MS. Vitamin B_{12} is important for maintaining normal nerve function, and low levels of vitamin B_{12} may produce injury to the optic nerves and the spinal cord, two components of the nervous system that also are damaged in MS. However, this does not mean that vitamin B_{12} deficiency and MS are similar diseases.

It is sometimes assumed that people with neurologic diseases such as MS should take vitamin B_{12} supplements because vitamin B_{12} deficiency causes neurologic injury. This is not a logical argument. Low levels of vitamin B_{12} are harmful to nerves, but no evidence suggests that high levels are any better for nerve function than are normal levels. Of note, a small study of six people with progressive MS found that massive doses of vitamin B_{12} taken for 6 months did not produce any improvement in disability (5).

In another study of 138 people with MS, treatment was for 24 weeks using vitamin B_{12} alone or with the *Cari Loder regime*, which uses vitamin B_{12} along with two other compounds, phenylalanine and lofepramine (6,7). After 2 weeks of treatment, both groups showed mild neurological improvement. Those treated with the *Cari Loder regime* had mild additional neurological improvement and symptom relief. The significance of the relatively small treatment effects seen in this study is not clear.

Studies of vitamin B_{12} levels in people with MS have produced variable results. It is clear from these studies that the majority of people with MS have normal vitamin B_{12} levels. There may be a small subgroup of people with MS who have low vitamin B_{12} levels. The cause for this low level in some people with MS is not known.

People with suspected MS should be evaluated for vitamin B_{12} deficiency, because of the rare association of vitamin B_{12} deficiency and MS. Vitamin B_{12} levels should be evaluated through blood testing ordered by a physician or other health care provider. If the vitamin B_{12} level is normal, no further vitamin B_{12} testing is required, and vitamin B_{12} supplements are not necessary. If the vitamin B_{12} level is low, further testing may be needed, and vitamin B_{12} injections or pills may be indicated. The usual treatment for vitamin B_{12} deficiency is monthly injections of the vitamin. Oral treatment also may be possible. Lifetime therapy is often necessary, and follow-up vitamin B_{12} testing may be indicated on an intermittent basis. Although vitamin B_{12} supplements are generally well tolerated, they may rarely cause itching, diarrhea, and rashes.

Other B Vitamins

For unstated or illogical reasons, B vitamin supplementation sometimes is recommended for MS. The B vitamins include vitamin B_1 (thiamine), vitamin B_2 (riboflavin), vitamin B_3 (niacin), vitamin B_5 (pantothenic acid), vitamin B_6 (pyridoxine), vitamin B_7 (biotin), vitamin B_{12} (cobalamin), and folate (or folic acid).

B vitamins are sometimes recommended because they play an important role in the functioning of both the immune system and the nervous system. It is recognized that deficiencies of several of the B vitamins can produce serious disorders of the immune system and the nervous system. However, because deficiencies produce abnormalities, it should not then be assumed that high intake amounts are better than normal intake levels.

Folic acid may play a role in regulating immune function. Research shows no consistent findings of decreased levels of folic acid in people with MS. In addition, no clinical studies demonstrate that supplements of folic acid are beneficial for MS. For people who take methotrexate, a chemotherapy agent occasionally used to treat MS, the toxic effects of the drug may be decreased by taking folic acid supplements.

At this time, no research evidence demonstrates that people with MS in general benefit from B vitamin supplementation. As noted in the section on vitamin B_{12}, a small subgroup of people with MS have vitamin B_{12} deficiency and should be treated. High doses of the other B vitamins should be avoided. In particular, excessive doses of vitamin B_6 (pyridoxine) and vitamin B_3 (niacin) should be avoided:

■   More than 50 milligrams daily of vitamin B_6 (pyridoxine) may produce nerve injury. This may result in numbness and tingling in the hands and feet, which is similar to symptoms that may be experienced with MS. A theoretical risk also exists of immune stimulation with high doses of vitamin B_6.

■ Greater than 35 milligrams of vitamin B_3 (niacin) daily may produce flushing, nausea, liver injury, and increased blood sugar levels.

Multivitamins

Multivitamins frequently are taken by people with MS. Multivitamin preparations contain variable types and amounts of vitamins and minerals.

No rigorous clinical studies have examined the benefits or safety of multivitamin use in MS. Studies in the elderly indicate that multivitamin preparations may stimulate the immune system. This type of stimulation may theoretically be harmful for MS. However, the significance of this immune-system effect for a disease process such as MS is not clear at this time.

Multivitamins may be particularly beneficial for those with special nutritional needs, such as:

■ Women who are pregnant or are trying to become pregnant
■ People on restricted diets
■ Strict vegetarians
■ People with gastrointestinal conditions or other nutrient-depleting diseases, such as cancer or diabetes

Standard multivitamin supplements should typically contain 18 nutrients—11 vitamins and 7 minerals:

■ Vitamins—Vitamins A, B_1 (thiamine), B_2 (riboflavin), B_3 (niacin), B_6 (pyridoxine), B_{12}, C, D, E, K; folic acid
■ Minerals—Calcium, copper, magnesium, phosphorous, potassium, selenium, zinc

A multivitamin preparation is important for people with MS who have an inadequate intake of vitamins and minerals. For people with MS who have an adequate diet, the benefits of multivitamin preparations are not known. If multivitamins are taken, it is important to review the amount of each vitamin and mineral in a preparation. Obviously, toxic doses should be avoided (see Table 43.2). Commercially available multivitamins do not generally contain toxic doses of any compounds, but some high-potency "designer" multivitamins may contain high doses of particular vitamins or minerals. For people with MS, it may be logical, although of no proven benefit, to use low doses of potentially immune-stimulating vitamins and minerals, including vitamin A, vitamin C, vitamin E, selenium, and zinc. Low daily doses of these vitamins and minerals are:

- Vitamin A—5,000 IU or less
- Vitamin C—90 to 120 milligrams or less
- Vitamin E—100 IU or less
- Selenium—20 to 55 micrograms or less
- Zinc—10 to 15 milligrams or less

Minerals

Calcium

Calcium supplements are sometimes recommended for MS, often for unstated reasons. Calcium supplements should be taken by people with inadequate dietary intakes of calcium. Also, calcium and vitamin D supplements are indicated for people with MS who have osteoporosis or risk factors for osteoporosis (see "Vitamin D and Calcium" in this chapter). No other clear uses are apparent for calcium supplements in MS. It should be noted that calcium interferes with iron absorption; consequently, calcium and iron supplements should not be taken together.

Selenium

Selenium is a mineral sometimes recommended for MS. This recommendation may be based on its known antioxidant activity or on studies suggesting that people with MS have low selenium levels. It is not clear that selenium is a reasonable supplement for people with MS.

As noted in the section on antioxidant vitamins, antioxidant compounds may have several beneficial effects on MS. However, most antioxidant compounds, including selenium, activate the immune system, and this immune-system stimulation may conceivably worsen MS. In fact, in one study of animals with EAE, an experimental form of MS, selenium supplementation *worsened* the disease course and *increased* the mortality rate. Also, the severity of the disease was the same for animals fed low-selenium and normal-selenium diets. The results of this study suggest that selenium supplementation may actually be harmful for people with MS.

The influence of selenium on MS itself is not known because no large study has ever directly examined the effects of selenium supplements on people with the disease. One small study found that treatment with selenium and several antioxidant vitamins did not produce adverse effects in people with MS. However, this study was too small (18 people) and too short in duration (5 weeks) to be definitive (1).

Because of the limited information about selenium, it is not clear whether selenium supplementation in MS produces beneficial effects, harmful effects, or no effects at all. It may be most reasonable for people with MS to avoid selenium supplements until more information is available. Selenium may be obtained in the diet from seafood, meat, and whole grains. If supplements are taken, it may be best to take low doses, such as 20 to 55 micrograms or less daily. High doses (greater than 400 micrograms) should be avoided because they may activate the immune system and may produce fatigue, nausea, dizziness, hair loss, tooth decay, and other problems.

Zinc

Zinc supplementation sometimes is recommended for MS. In fact, zinc phosphate was one of the earliest recommended therapies for MS. Zinc phosphate was used in the 1880s as a treatment by colleagues of Jean-Martin Charcot, a French neurologist who played a major role in defining MS as a disease. At this time, no clear reasons exist for people with MS to take zinc supplements.

Zinc may have beneficial effects on the common cold. Some, but not all, studies indicate that zinc lozenges shorten the duration of the common cold. Zinc lozenges do not appear to be effective for preventing the common cold. The possible therapeutic effect of zinc is of potential importance to people with MS because the common cold and other viral infections may trigger MS attacks.

Zinc supplements are also sometimes recommended in MS because zinc is involved in the chemical pathway of polyunsaturated fatty acids, as discussed in the chapter on "Diet and Fatty Acid Supplements". This chemical pathway has been implicated in MS. However, it is not known if the pathway is indeed involved in MS, and it is not known whether zinc supplements are necessary for this pathway to function normally.

It is important to recognize that zinc may actually *stimulate* the immune system. Zinc activates several different immune cells, including macrophages and T cells. In fact, zinc supplements appear to increase the amount of brain inflammation in EAE, an animal model of MS. This suggests that supplements in humans may worsen MS.

A possible toxic role for zinc was suggested by a report of a relatively high occurrence of MS in a zinc-related industry in New York. Blood levels of zinc were increased in people in this facility. Studies of zinc levels in other MS populations have produced inconsistent results: Some studies show high levels, but other studies indicate low levels. A *deficiency* of zinc produced *benefits* in a mouse model of lupus, an autoimmune disorder like MS. This finding is consistent with immune stimulation by zinc.

A high intake of zinc actually may cause a serious neurological disorder, known as *copper-deficiency myelopathy*, that may mimic MS. Multiple causes are known for this disorder, which has been recognized recently. One cause is a high intake of zinc that leads to high blood levels of zinc and low blood levels of copper. In this condition, as in MS, abnormalities occur in the spinal cord, and people may experience difficulties with walking and sensation.

Immune-system activation by zinc could worsen MS. Given the fact that zinc has unclear benefits and that it may potentially stimulate the immune system, it is reasonable for people with MS to avoid zinc supplements or to use low doses of supplements—such as 10 to 15 milligrams or less daily.

Other Minerals

A whole variety of minerals sometimes are recommended for people with MS. Some studies indicate that people with MS have low levels of specific minerals, such as magnesium, zinc, and copper. The meaning of these results is not known. Before 1935, some recommended therapies for MS actually involved supplements of minerals, including antimony, arsenic, mercury, potassium bromide, potassium iodide, and thorium. At this time, no published clinical studies demonstrate a definite therapeutic effect in MS using supplements of these or other minerals, including chromium, cobalt, copper, iodine, magnesium, molybdenum, phosphorus, potassium (in various forms), and vanadium. Finally, gold or silver supplements have been recommended for MS. These are of no proven benefit, and silver supplements may actually produce serious toxic effects.

Other Supplements

5-HTP

5-HTP (5-hydroxytryptophan) is a type of chemical known as an amino acid. It is chemically similar to another amino acid, tryptophan. 5-HTP may be effective for treating depression. Tryptophan itself was sold for this use in the past. Unfortunately, contaminated batches produced a serious condition, *eosinophilia-myalgia syndrome*. Although this condition was thought to be due to contaminants known as *peak X*, and *peak X* is not present in some 5-HTP preparations, other compounds may be involved. Due to these uncertainties and the fact that 5-HTP may contain some of the same contaminants as tryptophan, it is reasonable to avoid 5-HTP until more information is available.

Acetyl-L-Carnitine

Acetyl-L-carnitine, sometimes referred to as *ALCAR*, is a compound that has been studied in people with memory difficulties and fatigue. (Note: *L-carnitine* is a different compound.) Acetyl-L-carnitine may improve memory in people with Alzheimer's disease and other memory disorders, and it also may decrease fatigue in people with a variety of conditions.

Due to its possible fatigue-relieving effects, acetyl-L-carnitine was evaluated in a study of 36 people with MS (8). The effects of a standard MS fatigue medication, amantadine (Symmetrel), were compared with those of acetyl-L-carnitine over a 3-month period. This small study found a significant decrease in one measure of fatigue (the *FSS* or *Fatigue Severity Scale*) with the use of acetyl-L-carnitine but not with amantadine. Using another measure of fatigue (the *FIS* or *Fatigue Impact Scale*), neither therapy produced significant effects. These findings suggest that acetyl-L-carnitine may be effective for MS-related fatigue—larger studies are needed to determine if this therapy is definitely effective.

Acetyl-L-carnitine usually is well tolerated. In the MS study of acetyl-L-carnitine, one person discontinued acetyl-L-carnitine due to side effects, which were insomnia and anxiety. In that same study, five people discontinued amantadine because of adverse effects, which included nausea and dizziness. In other studies, it has been found that acetyl-L-carnitine may cause nausea, vomiting, and agitation. Acetyl-L-carnitine is not known to interact with any medications. It has been recommended that people taking acetyl-L-carnitine have intermittent blood tests, including complete blood count (CBC) and tests of liver and kidney function. Trials with acetyl-L-carnitine have used doses of 1,500 to 4,000 milligrams daily, which is usually divided into two or three doses. In the MS study of acetyl-L-carnitine, 1,000 milligrams was administered twice daily.

Alpha-Lipoic Acid

Alpha-lipoic acid is an antioxidant compound. Like the antioxidant vitamins, alpha-lipoic acid acts to decrease the damage produced by free radicals. Alpha-lipoic acid normally is present in the *mitochondria*, the energy-producing parts of the body's cells.

Alpha-lipoic acid may have relevance to neurological disorders, including MS. Encouraging results with alpha-lipoic acid have been obtained in animal and human studies by Dr. Dennis Bourdette and others at Oregon Health Sciences University (OHSU) (9,10). In EAE, the animal model of MS, alpha-lipoic acid deceases the severity of the disease. This appears to be due to the ability of alpha-lipoic acid to inhibit the movement of immune cells from the blood into the central nervous system. In a small study in people with MS, alpha-lipoic acid was generally well tolerated and appeared to inhibit two proteins involved in immune-cell movement into the central nervous system (*MMP-9* and *sICAM-1*). Further studies of alpha-lipoic acid are underway at OHSU.

Some studies indicate that alpha-lipoic acid may be helpful for diabetes itself and also for a diabetes-associated form of nerve injury known as *polyneuropathy*. Studies of alpha-lipoic acid in other neurologic conditions are currently being conducted. Limited information is available about the safety of alpha-lipoic acid, especially for long-term use and for use in people with MS.

Amino Acids

Amino acids are chemicals used to synthesize proteins in the body. Mixtures of specific amino acids known as *branched-chain amino acids* sometimes are recommended for MS. There is no evidence that people with MS are deficient in amino acids or that amino acid therapy is beneficial for MS. Branched-chain amino acids do not appear to improve physical performance in athletes. Importantly, high doses (greater than 20 grams daily) may produce fatigue by increasing the amount of ammonia in the blood.

Specific amino acids have been studied for their effects on MS symptoms, MS itself, or the animal model of MS; these include 5-HTP, tryptophan, and threonine. See the relevant sections for descriptions of these compounds.

Androstenedione

Androstenedione became well known to the public after the baseball player Mark McGwire acknowledged that he used it in 1998. Androstenedione is a hormone sold as a dietary supplement. In the body, it is converted to testosterone, the male sex hormone. Androstenedione is of potential interest to people with MS because it is claimed to increase strength and energy.

However, clinical studies do not support its claimed benefits. Androstenedione does not increase muscle strength or muscle size. Androstenedione does not appear to increase testosterone levels on a long-term basis. It does increase estrogen levels, which may increase the risk of conditions and cancers that are sensitive to this hormone, including endometriosis, uterine fibroids, and cancers of the breast, uterus, ovaries, and prostate. Androstenedione decreases levels of HDL, the "good" form of cholesterol, and may thereby increase the risk of heart disease and stroke. Multiple other possible side effects may occur with androstenedione.

Androstenedione should be avoided because of its unclear benefits and its multiple possible side effects.

Caffeine

Caffeine is of potential interest because MS may cause fatigue, and caffeine may improve mental alertness. Caffeine is available in tablet form as a dietary supplement. The use of these tablets, coffee, and other caffeine-containing herbs is discussed in the "Herbs" chapter.

Calcium EAP

In the early 1960s, Dr. Hans Nieper, a German physician, developed a compound known as calcium EAP. It is also known as calcium-2-aminoethyl phosphate, calcium AEP, and calcium orotate. Thousands of people have apparently been treated with this compound. Most information about calcium EAP is available only from literature by Dr. Nieper (who died in 1998) or organizations affiliated with him.

Calcium EAP is one component of an approach to MS referred to as the *Nieper regimen*. It is believed that calcium EAP allows necessary chemicals to interact with nerve cells and protects nerve cells from injury by the immune system and by toxins. Several other principles underlie the Nieper regimen, including claims that milk and several minerals (chlorine, chromium, fluoride, platinum) play an important role in MS.

The Nieper program recommends calcium EAP treatment along with other measures. Calcium EAP initially is given intravenously in a dosage of 500 milligrams per day for 5 days per week. It is then given long-term as a pill or as an every-other-day intravenous dose of 400 milligrams. Other recommendations include steroid treatment with prednisone (5 to 8 milligrams daily); vitamin and mineral supplements (some at high doses), including selenium and vitamins C, D, and E; avoidance of bright sunlight, alcohol, milk and milk products, evening primrose oil, aluminum, fluoride, and drinks that contain phosphoric acid or quinine; avoidance of water in the environment by not using waterbeds and hiring a dowser to be certain no underground water exists near one's bedroom; and consumption of olive oil and raw food because of their *Kirlian positivity*.

No well-designed clinical trials of calcium EAP have been published. Calcium EAP was first used in Europe in 1964 and in the United States in 1972. A document written by Dr. Nieper in 1968 describes the treatment of 167 people with MS. Beneficial effects were observed in 46 percent with mild disease, 33 percent with moderate disease, and 16 percent with severe disease. The overall benefit was 32 percent. Importantly, no placebo group was used in this study. Other literature by Dr. Nieper claims benefits in 85 to 90 percent of people with MS. Overall, no well-designed studies exist to determine whether calcium EAP is beneficial for people with MS.

The safety of calcium EAP has not been established. Of concern is a 1990 report in which a 53-year-old woman with MS had an abrupt cessation of heart and lung function (cardiopulmonary arrest) during intravenous administration of calcium EAP. She was resuscitated and subsequently developed serious kidney, liver, and bleeding complications.

By Dr. Nieper's account, in animal studies, 1 in 10 animals develop kidney stones, females gain weight, and males become aggressive. Apparently, these side effects have not been observed in people. Some people treated with calcium EAP develop headaches and chills.

In conclusion, there is no rigorous published evidence that calcium EAP has beneficial effects. Calcium EAP may be very costly. One report documents serious complications with intravenous use, and no studies document the safety of long-term use.

Coenzyme Q10

Coenzyme Q10 is also known as *CoQ10* or *ubiquinone*. Like some vitamins, coenzyme Q10 is an antioxidant that may decrease free radical damage. Also, coenzyme Q10 may improve the function of mitochondria, the energy-producing components of the body's cells.

Coenzyme Q10 use has been claimed to produce many different health benefits. Some of these claims are not justified. Coenzyme Q10 may have applications to neurological disorders, especially those that are thought to involve free-radical damage or impaired function of the mitochondria. Coenzyme Q10 may be beneficial for several heart problems, including a condition known as congestive heart failure.

No large published studies have evaluated coenzyme Q10 in people with MS. As for the antioxidant vitamins (see earlier in this section), coenzyme Q10 may have beneficial effects on MS. However, like many antioxidant compounds, coenzyme Q10 stimulates T cells and macrophages, two types of immune cells, and may therefore adversely affect MS or antagonize the effects of MS medications such as interferons (Avonex, Betaseron, Rebif), glatiramer acetate (Copaxone), mitoxantrone (Novantrone), and natalizumab (Tysabri).

The effects on MS of antioxidant supplements such as coenzyme Q10 are not known. If antioxidants are taken, vitamins A, C, or E are more economical than coenzyme Q10. Coenzyme Q10 may decrease the effect of blood-thinning medication (warfarin or Coumadin). High doses of coenzyme Q10 (more than 300 milligrams daily) may cause mild liver toxicity.

Creatine

Creatine is a supplement claimed to increase muscle strength and increase body mass. In addition, it may have a protective effect on nerves. Both of these possible effects are relevant to MS.

Creatine is made in the liver, kidneys, and pancreas. It is involved in generating energy for muscle cells and other cells in the body. Creatine is available as a dietary supplement and may be obtained in the diet by eating meat and fish.

Limited clinical studies have been done on creatine. In healthy people, creatine supplements may improve performance for brief, high-intensity exercises. In one study of 16 people with MS, creatine supplements did not improve high-intensity exercise ability or increase the muscle stores of creatine (11). In people with diseases of the muscles (such as muscular dystrophy), limited studies indicate that creatine may increase strength, decrease muscle fatigue, and improve exercise capacity.

Creatine usually is well tolerated when used in appropriate doses. Rarely, creatine may cause kidney failure, especially in those with known kidney disease. Other possible side effects of creatine include stomach pain, nausea, diarrhea, weight gain, dehydration, and muscle cramping.

Dehydroepiandrosterone (DHEA)

DHEA (dehydroepiandrosterone) is a hormone available as a dietary supplement. It is marketed as an antiaging compound and as a "miracle cure" for many medical conditions. Claimed benefits of DHEA of potential interest to people with MS include improvement in fatigue, sex drive, and mood.

DHEA is a naturally occurring steroid hormone produced by the adrenal glands. DHEA may be important for aging because blood levels of DHEA generally decrease significantly as people get older.

Studies on DHEA have not demonstrated definite benefits. DHEA may have beneficial effects on aging skin, erectile dysfunction, and menopausal symptoms. DHEA does not appear to improve muscle strength or cognitive ability.

Limited information is available about the effects of DHEA on immune system–related diseases such as MS. In the animal model of MS, DHEA appears to have an anti-inflammatory effect and to decrease the severity of the disease. However, in other studies, DHEA appears to activate T cells, immune cells that are already excessively active in MS. This effect raises a theoretical risk for DHEA use in MS. In another autoimmune disease, lupus, DHEA may be beneficial in the mouse model of the disease and for people with the disease. Additional research on the effects of DHEA in MS and other immunological diseases is needed.

DHEA has multiple possible adverse effects. It may cause liver injury. Other side effects include acne, hair loss, voice deepening, fatigue, altered menstruation, abdominal pain, hypertension, and increased risk of some hormone-sensitive cancers, including breast, endometrial, and prostate cancer. The safety of long-term DHEA use has not been established.

No strong reason exists for people with MS to take DHEA supplements. No definite benefits are associated with its use. Although encouraging results with DHEA have been noted in the animal model of MS, DHEA also carries a theoretical risk as a result of immune stimulation, and it may cause multiple adverse effects, especially in women.

Germanium

Germanium is a compound sometimes recommended as a therapy for MS. However, no studies of germanium in MS have been done, and it may cause significant side effects, including kidney failure, weakness, nerve injury, anemia, and death. There have been 31 reports of death or kidney failure related to germanium use.

Glucosamine

Glucosamine is a dietary supplement that appears to be effective for treating arthritis. Glucosamine mildly suppresses the immune system—it appears to decrease the activity of the inflammatory component of the immune system (*Th1* response) and increase the activity of the anti-inflammatory component (*Th2* response). In EAE, the animal model of MS, glucosamine decreases disease severity (12). These findings are encouraging. Further animal studies and, if indicated, human studies are needed to understand the possible effects of glucosamine on MS. Glucosamine generally is well tolerated. It may cause mild side effects, such as gastrointestinal complaints, headache, and drowsiness.

Inosine

Inosine is a compound that is converted in the body to uric acid. Uric acid has antioxidant effects. Promising results have been obtained with uric acid treatment of the animal model of MS (13). In a small study of 11 people with MS, inosine treatment increased blood levels of uric acid and was associated with clinical improvement in three people (14). Further studies of inosine are underway. Episodes of gout are caused by high blood levels of uric acid. As a result, raising blood levels of uric acid with inosine may provoke gout attacks. The safety of long-term inosine use is not known.

Lecithin

Lecithin, which contains phosphatidylcholine, is a supplement sometimes recommended for MS. Phosphatidylcholine is involved in several body processes, and it is a major component of cell membranes. Supplements of lecithin are made from soybean oil. At this time, there are no studies to indicate that lecithin therapy is beneficial to people with MS. Lecithin is usually well tolerated—it has been classified as Generally Regarded as Safe (GRAS) by the FDA. Lecithin may cause diarrhea, nausea, and abdominal pain, especially when used in high doses (greater than 20 grams daily).

Melatonin

Melatonin is a hormone produced in the *pineal gland*, a small gland in the brain. Melatonin is involved in regulating *circadian rhythms*, the regular daily cycles of the body, such as sleeping and waking. Blood levels of melatonin are high at night and low during the day.

Many therapeutic benefits have been claimed for melatonin. Most studies have evaluated its effects on sleeping problems. For insomnia, some, but not all, clinical investigations have shown a therapeutic effect with melatonin. Melatonin also may be effective for the prevention of jet lag.

A possible role of melatonin in causing MS has been proposed. In one study, high blood levels of melatonin were associated with a later age of onset of the disease and a shorter duration of the disease. The significance of these findings in relation to melatonin causing MS or the effect of taking melatonin supplements on MS is not known

People with MS should be aware that melatonin may activate the immune system. The effects of melatonin on the immune system are not fully understood. However, specific immune cells called T cells have sites to which melatonin attaches, and some studies have shown that melatonin stimulates T cells. Paradoxically, in the animal model of MS, one study showed that melatonin improved the disease, whereas another study showed that luzindole, a compound that blocks the effects of melatonin, was also therapeutic—clearly, more work is needed in this area. Due to its immune-stimulating effects, it has been proposed that melatonin may worsen another autoimmune disease, rheumatoid arthritis, but be beneficial for AIDS and cancer.

In summary, melatonin may be helpful for insomnia and jet lag. However, it carries a theoretical risk for people with MS because it may stimulate the immune system. Until more information is available, it would be reasonable for people with MS to avoid melatonin. If melatonin is used by people with MS, high doses and long-term use should probably be avoided.

Oligomeric Proanthocyanidins

Oligomeric proanthocyanidins (OPCs) are antioxidant compounds. They are one of the main components in several antioxidant supplements, including pycnogenol and grape seed extract. As noted in the sections on these substances, it is not clear that the antioxidant effects of OPCs are beneficial to people with MS. Furthermore, they are more expensive than conventional antioxidant vitamins.

S-adenosylmethionine (SAMe)

SAMe (S-adenosylmethionine; also known as Sammy) is a supplement claimed to be an effective treatment for multiple medical conditions. SAMe is a naturally occurring compound involved in fundamental biochemical reactions called *methylation reactions*. These reactions also involve vitamin B_{12} and folic acid. SAMe has been commercially available for years in European countries, including Germany, Italy, and Spain. SAMe became available as a dietary supplement in the United States in the spring of 1999.

Multiple therapeutic effects have been attributed to SAMe. Multiple studies indicate that SAMe reduces depression, which is relevant because depression may occur with MS. The mechanism by which SAMe may produce its antidepressant effect is not known. SAMe also may be effective for liver disease, fibromyalgia, a form of arthritis known as osteoarthritis, and a spinal cord condition that occurs in people with AIDS.

It has been claimed that SAMe may be a treatment for MS. This claim is based on several observations of uncertain significance. First, a small subgroup of people with MS have vitamin B_{12} deficiency. Because SAMe and vitamin B_{12} are involved in similar chemical reactions, it is proposed that SAMe is beneficial for MS. In addition, SAMe sometimes is used to treat some rare genetic diseases that produce injury to the nerve cells in a manner somewhat similar to the nerve damage produced by MS. However, these arguments for SAMe treatment of MS are not well grounded. There is no evidence that abnormalities in vitamin B_{12} or SAMe play a major role in MS, and levels of SAMe are normal in the spinal fluid of people with MS.

SAMe is claimed to be a potential treatment for other neurologic disorders, including Parkinson's disease, Alzheimer's disease, and epilepsy. Current research does not support the use of SAMe for these conditions.

In general, SAMe appears to be well tolerated. In clinical studies, no major toxicity has been reported in 22,000 people treated with SAMe. Minor side effects are nausea, vomiting, diarrhea, constipation, dry mouth, mild insomnia, dizziness, and anxiety. SAMe should not be used with antidepressant medications. SAMe may increase the adverse as well as therapeutic effects of steroids. SAMe may decrease the effectiveness of the Parkinson's disease medication levodopa.

Depression is a serious condition, and anyone who feels that he or she is depressed should be evaluated by a physician. Treatment with SAMe—or any other antidepressant compound—should be done in conjunction with a physician. In clinical studies of depression, the daily dose of SAMe has been 400 to 1,600 milligrams.

Threonine

Threonine is an amino acid that has been studied in people with MS who have muscle stiffness or spasticity. In the body, threonine is converted to another chemical, glycine, which could decrease spasticity. Research suggests that threonine improves stiffness as measured by formal clinical testing. However, this effect is so mild that it is not noticeable to people taking the compound or to examining clinicians. Thus, threonine does not appear to be effective enough to use for MS-associated spasticity.

Tryptophan

Tryptophan is a compound known as an amino acid. It is present in many plants and animals; this is the chemical sometimes claimed to produce the fatigue that occurs after a turkey dinner. The chemical breakdown products of tryptophan are thought to play a role in inflammatory processes. A recent study of the animal model of MS evaluated the effects of a synthetic compound similar to the breakdown products of tryptophan (15). This compound is known as *3,4 DAA*, which is a shortened notation for *N-(3,4,-dimethoxycinnamoyl) anthranilic acid)*. 3,4 DAA decreases the production of inflammatory immune cells. In addition, it decreases the severity of disease in the animal model of MS. Interestingly, the structure of this compound is similar to that of two drugs, *linomid and laquinomod*, that have produced promising results in MS-related animal and human studies. Further research with 3,4 DAA and related tryptophan compounds is needed.

Conclusion

People with MS should be cautious in their use of supplements. Among vitamins, vitamin D may be underutilized for osteoporosis. Antioxidant vitamins (and other supplements with antioxidant effects) have produced promising results in animal studies and limited human trials. Recommendations about antioxidant supplement use cannot be made until further research is conducted in this area. Vitamin C does not appear to be effective for the prevention or treatment of urinary tract infections. A small subgroup of people with MS may have vitamin B_{12} deficiency and should be treated with vitamin B_{12} supplements. It is reasonable for people with MS to avoid multivitamins containing high doses of possibly immune-stimulating vitamins and minerals.

Among other supplements, SAMe may be effective as an antidepressant. Creatine may improve muscle strength, but it produced negative results in a small study in people with MS. In one study, acetyl-L-carnitine produced promising effects on fatigue in people with MS. Caffeine may also conceivably improve MS fatigue, but this has not been formally studied. Two compounds, glucosamine and a tryptophan-related compound, have produced therapeutic effects in the animal model of MS. Calcium EAP is expensive and has no well-documented benefits for MS. Selenium, zinc, DHEA, and melatonin may activate the immune system and thus should be avoided or used in low doses for limited periods. Androstenedione may be harmful and has no clear benefits.

Additional Readings

Books

Bowling AC, Stewart TS. *Dietary Supplements and Multiple Sclerosis: A Health Professional's Guide.* New York: Demos Medical Publishing, 2004.

Fetrow CW, Avila JR. *Professional's Handbook of Complementary and Alternative Medicines.* Philadelphia: Lippincott, Williams, & Wilkins, 2004.

Fragakis AS. *The Health Professional's Guide to Popular Dietary Supplements.* The American Dietetic Association, 2003.

Jellin JM, Batz F, Hitchens K, et al. *Natural Medicines Comprehensive Database.* Stockton, CA: Therapeutic Research Faculty, 2006.

Polman CH, Thompson AJ, Murray TJ, Bowling AC, Noseworthy JH. *Multiple Sclerosis: The Guide to Treatment and Management.* New York: Demos Medical Publishing, 2006.

Ulbricht CE, Basch EM, eds. *Natural Standard Herb and Supplement Reference: Evidence-Based Clinical Reviews.* St. Louis: Elsevier-Mosby, 2005.

Journal Articles

Anon. Spin the bottle. How to pick a multivitamin. *Nutrition Action Healthletter* 2003;Jan–Feb:3–9.

Anon. Multivitamins: what to avoid, how to choose. *Cons Reports* 2006;Feb:19–20.

Mai J, Sorensen PS, Hansen JC. High dose antioxidant supplementation to MS patients. *Biol Trace Elem Res* 1990;24:109–117.

Platten M, Ho PP, Yousseff S, et al. Treatment of autoimmune neuroinflammation with a synthetic tryptophan metabolite. *Science* 2005;310:850–855.

Tomassini V, Pozzilli C, Onesti E, et al. Comparison of the effects of acetyl-L-carnitine and amantadine for the treatment of fatigue in multiple sclerosis: results of a pilot, randomised, double-blind, crossover trial. *J Neurol Sci* 2004;218:103–108.

Van Meeteren ME, Teunissen CE, Dijkstra CD, et al. Antioxidants and polyunsaturated fatty acids in multiple sclerosis. *Eur J Clin Nutr* 2005;59:1347–1361.

Wingerchuk DM, Lesaux J, Rice GPA, et al. A pilot study of oral calcitriol (1,25-dihydroxyvitamin D3) for relapsing-remitting multiple sclerosis. *J Neurol Neurosurg Psych* 2005;76:1294–1296.

Yadav V, Marracci G, Lovera J, et al. Lipoic acid in multiple sclerosis: a pilot study. *Mult Scler* 2005;11:159–165.

Zhang GX, Yu S, Gran B, et al. Glucosamine abrogates the acute phase of experimental autoimmune encephalomyelitis by induction of Th2 response. *J Neuroimmunol* 2005;175:7202–7208.

44

Yoga

Yoga was developed thousands of years ago in India. It is related to the Hindu religion, and was created as a spiritual practice. Yoga means "union" in Sanskrit and is believed to unite the mind, body, and spirit.

Treatment Method

Yoga takes many different forms. One of the more popular forms in the United States is *hatha yoga*. Three main components of yoga are breathing, movement, and posture. A series of body postures and movements, known as *asanas*, are performed. Deep, slow breathing is done in conjunction with the body movements. Specific breathing exercises, referred to as *pranayama*, also are done. Different types of yoga have different levels of exercise intensity and posture difficulty. In addition to these physical activities, yoga may include meditation, ethical guidelines, and diet recommendations.

In contrast to popular belief, the primary aim of yoga is not to attempt to assume difficult, contorted postures. People who are not able to maintain postures may still perform yoga. Postures in the standing or seated position are made easier by the use of "props," such as straps and wooden blocks. Yoga may be practiced by people who have severe arm and leg weakness. In this situation, emphasis is placed on head and shoulder movement, breathing exercises, and meditation. On the surface, this limited program may not appear to be yoga, but it does in fact focus on the same elements as more conventional yoga techniques.

Studies in MS and Other Conditions

Despite its popularity, only a limited number of research studies have been undertaken with yoga. Unfortunately, many of them are small or have significant flaws. The effects of yoga on symptoms observed in multiple sclerosis

(MS) have undergone limited investigation. One well-designed study evaluated the effects of yoga on MS symptoms (1). In this study, 69 people with MS were treated for six months with a conventional exercise program, yoga, or no intervention. Those treated with yoga or conventional exercise showed decreased fatigue. No effect on mood or cognitive function was noted with the use of yoga or conventional exercise. In other studies, anxiety and stress have been reduced with yoga—this effect may be long-lasting. Several studies in the general population indicate that yoga may relieve depression. People with pain, including headaches and low back pain, may benefit from yoga. Some reports document decreased muscle stiffness with yoga, but this has not been formally studied.

An active yoga program for people with MS in southern California has been developed by Eric Small and the southern California chapter of the National Multiple Sclerosis Society. Small, who has MS, studied yoga in India and England. He began practicing yoga shortly after he was diagnosed with the disease. His disease has been relatively mild over the course of 40 years. He has adapted classic yoga poses so that they can be done by people with significant physical disabilities. Many of the students who have participated in his program have required the use of walkers or wheelchairs. In interviews with people in his program, beneficial effects have been noted in both emotional and physical functioning. People have described improvements in depression, concentration, memory, sense of well-being, breathing, walking steadiness, strength, and stiffness.

Yoga has been investigated in other diseases. In asthma, yoga has been associated with decreased medication use, increased lung function, positive attitude, and relaxation. It may decrease joint pain and improve joint movements for people with arthritis. Yoga may be helpful for diabetes and may decrease heart rate and blood pressure.

Side Effects

Yoga usually is not associated with any significant adverse effects. However, yoga involving difficult postures or vigorous exercise should be performed with caution by those with the following conditions:

- Pregnancy
- Fatigue, sensitivity to heat, or impaired balance
- Significant lung, heart, and bone conditions
- Significant spine problems, such as herniated discs
- Recent surgery

If meditation is considered, people with psychiatric disorders should discuss this therapy with their psychiatrist (see the chapter on "Meditation"). As with all forms of complementary and alternative medicine (CAM), yoga should not be used in place of conventional medicine, especially for trying to control the underlying disease process or significant MS-related symptoms.

Practical Information

Yoga may be performed in groups or individually. Yoga techniques may be learned in classes, which are about 60 minutes in length. Group classes cost between $15 and $30, and private sessions are $25 to $35 per hour. Benefiting from yoga requires an ongoing commitment; several hours per week over weeks to months generally are required.

Yoga classes often are available through recreation centers, the YMCA, and schools. A listing of yoga teachers is available each year in the July/August issue of the *Yoga Journal* (2020 Milvia Street, Berkeley CA 94704 [510-486-2858]).

Pathways Exercise Video for People with Limited Mobility is a video showing yoga poses designed for people with MS. Information about the southern California yoga and MS program may be obtained from the southern California chapter of the National Multiple Sclerosis Society at www.nationalmssociety.org/CAL/home or 2440 S. Sepulveda Boulevard, #115, Los Angeles CA 90064 (800-344-4867 or 310-479-4456). General information on yoga is available from several yoga organizations:

■ The American Yoga Association (www.americanyogaassociation.org), P.O. Box 19986, Sarasota FL 34236 (941-927-4977)
■ International Association of Yoga Therapists (www.iayt.org) 115 South McCormick Street, Suite 3, Prescott AZ 86303 (928-541-0004)

Conclusion

Yoga is relatively inexpensive and generally safe. In MS, yoga has been shown to decrease fatigue. Although it has not been rigorously investigated, yoga also may improve depression, anxiety, pain, and spasticity.

Additional Readings

Books

Ernst E, ed. *The Desktop Guide to Complementary and Alternative Medicine: An Evidence-Based Approach*. Edinburgh: Mosby, 2001, pp. 76–78.

Navarra T. *The Encyclopedia of Complementary and Alternative Medicine*. New York: Checkmark Books. 2005, pp. 164–172.

Polman CH, Thompson AJ, Murray TJ, Bowling AC, Noseworthy JH. *Multiple Sclerosis: The Guide to Treatment and Management*. New York: Demos Medical Publishing, 2006, pp. 164–165.

Riley D. Hatha yoga and meditation for neurological conditions. In: Oken BS, ed. *Complementary Therapies in Neurology*. London: Parthenon Publishing, 2004, pp. 159–167.

Ross R. Yoga as a therapeutic modality. In: Weintraub MI, Micozzi MS, eds. *Alternative and Complementary Treatments in Neurologic Illness*. New York: Churchill Livingstone, 2001, pp. 75–92.

Journal Articles

Despres L. Yoga and MS. *Yoga J* July/August 1997;96–103.

Nayak NN, Shankar K. Yoga: a therapeutic approach. *Phys Med Rehabil Clin N Amer* 2004;15:783–798.

Oken BS, Kishiyama S, Zajdel D, et al. Randomized controlled trial of yoga and exercise in multiple sclerosis. *Neurol* 2004;62:2058–2064.

Pilkington K, Kirkwood G, Rampes H, et al. Yoga for depression: the research evidence. *J Affect Disord* 2005;89:13–24.

A Five-Step Approach:
Integrating Conventional
and Unconventional
Medicine

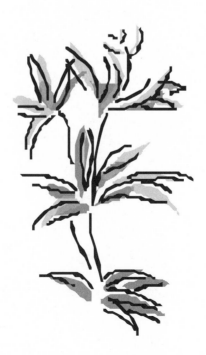

$\mathcal{M}$any conventional medical therapies are available for multiple sclerosis (MS) and, as reviewed in this book, a wide variety of possibly effective unconventional therapies also are available. For those who are interested in integrating conventional and unconventional therapies, how can all this information be used to best advantage? Is there a way to safely and wisely mix conventional and unconventional therapies?

It is possible to develop an approach to treating and managing multiple sclerosis (MS) that incorporates both conventional and unconventional approaches. This "integrative" approach ideally should have several features:

- Unbiased—Use evidence, not prejudices, to determine which therapies may be beneficial
- Individualized—Have flexibility in the approach so that it accounts for different personalities and orientations, and also accounts for MS having different effects on different people
- Broad-based—Aim to treat the underlying disease process (disease-modifying therapies) as well as MS-related symptoms (symptomatic therapies)

A Five-Step Approach

A broad-based approach that makes the best of both worlds by integrating conventional and unconventional approaches may be summarized in five steps:

- Step 1—Disease-modifying medications
- Step 2—Diet
- Step 3—Wellness approaches
- Step 4—Exercise
- Step 5—Integrative approach to symptom management

The remainder of this chapter will review these five steps in detail. Before considering these steps, it is important to realize that the information in this chapter is not intended as a recommendation for complementary and

247

alternative medicine (CAM) therapy. Any person with MS who is considering CAM therapy should strongly consider conventional medical therapy options and should thoroughly discuss any possible CAM therapies with his or her health care provider.

Precautions about CAM and MS should be kept in mind, as discussed in the introductory chapter. One precaution worth reiterating is that the information about nearly all forms of CAM is incomplete and, as a result, pursuing CAM presents uncertainties and risks. Best guesses can be made about CAM therapies, but it is possible that some therapies now presumed to be "probably safe" or "possibly effective" will eventually be classified as "definitely unsafe" or "definitely ineffective."

Many different unconventional therapies are mentioned briefly in this chapter. More detailed information about these therapies is presented in other chapters.

Step 1: Disease-Modifying Medications

At this time, the best available evidence for modifying the course of disease in MS is with one of the U.S. Food and Drug Administration (FDA)-approved disease-modifying medications. The commonly used medications are glatiramer acetate (Copaxone) and interferons (Avonex, Betaseron, Rebif). Other FDA-approved medications include natalizumab (Tysabri), and a chemotherapy medication, and mitoxantrone (Novantrone). Many other experimental medications and combinations of medications are undergoing clinical testing in MS.

Step 2: Diet

As outlined in Chapter 18, "Diets and Fatty Acid Supplements," a diet that is relatively low in saturated fat and enriched in polyunsaturated fatty acids may have mild disease-modifying effects in MS. The evidence in this area is suggestive but not definitive. Chapter 18 outlines approaches that may be taken with diet and dietary supplements.

Step 3: Wellness Approaches

"Wellness" is a term that is used so loosely and broadly that it sometimes loses its meaning. Chapter 2, "Placebos and Psychoneuroimmunology," discusses the placebo effect. Through a mind–body interaction, it is possible that a placebo response produces a disease-modifying effect in people with MS. A placebo response also may produce a symptomatic effect in MS. Trying to harness this placebo response is some of the intent of *wellness approaches*. A more descriptive term for these approaches would be personalized, empowering, and optimism- and hope-generating strategies.

The following are examples of approaches in this area and the people who may be particularly well-suited to these approaches:

- Spirituality and prayer, especially for those who are already spiritual
- Exercise, for those who feel empowered and relaxed when exercising
- Unconventional exercise, such as t'ai chi and yoga, for people who want to mix exercise and spirituality
- Relaxation methods, such as meditation and guided imagery, for those who feel relaxed when they are actually relaxing
- Alternative medical systems, such as traditional Chinese medicine and Ayurveda, may be especially well-suited for those who use conventional medicine but have some skepticism about it and want to have a practitioner who takes a completely different and unconventional approach
- Psychotherapy, for people with significant psychological issues

Step 4: Exercise

Exercise may provide beneficial effects for many different MS symptoms. Because of its many benefits, some form of exercise should be a component of a broad-based treatment plan. As explained in Chapter 20 on exercise, conventional and unconventional exercise programs are available. Conventional exercise programs may be developed with a physical therapist. Hydrotherapy, or water exercise, may be especially well-suited for people with MS who have leg weakness or walking difficulties. Unconventional exercise programs that may provide beneficial effects for those with MS include t'ai chi and yoga.

Step 5: Integrative Approach to Symptom Management

This step is the most complex. Often, MS treatment is focused on using either conventional therapies or a particular CAM approach to treat specific symptoms. In the integrative approach to symptom management, MS symptoms are considered in terms of all the approaches—conventional and unconventional—that may be reasonable. The use of these approaches, especially in combination, should be discussed with your health provider.

Anxiety and Stress

Anxiety and stress may occur in association with MS.

Conventional Medical Therapy

Conventional medical therapy in this area is often very effective. It typically involves the use of anti-anxiety medications and possibly psychotherapy.

Possibly Effective CAM Therapies

Anxiety and stress may be due to multiple causes, some of which may be the result of medical conditions. As a result, a physician should be consulted about the possible causes of anxiety before considering CAM therapies.

In general, CAM therapies for anxiety have not been studied extensively. The evidence supporting the use of conventional medical therapy, especially anti-anxiety medications, is much stronger than that for CAM therapy. CAM therapies that have yielded promising results are:

- Acupuncture
- Aromatherapy
- Ayurveda
- Biofeedback
- Exercise
- Feldenkrais
- Guided imagery
- Hypnosis
- Massage
- Meditation
- Music therapy
- Prayer
- Spirituality
- T'ai chi
- Therapeutic touch
- Yoga

Other CAM Therapies

Homeopathy generally is safe but is of uncertain effectiveness for anxiety. Kava kava should be avoided because of possible liver toxicity. Valerian is sometimes recommended for anxiety, but most studies of this herb have been for its use in insomnia.

Bladder Problems

MS may affect bladder function in several ways, including causing problems with storing urine, emptying urine, incontinence, and urinary tract infections (UTIs).

Conventional Therapy

Conventional therapy for these difficulties usually involves medications and lifestyle changes. Catheterization and surgical therapies may be indicated for more severe difficulties.

Possibly Effective CAM Therapies

People with recurrent UTIs should undergo a medical evaluation because it is important to determine the underlying cause. A CAM approach may be reasonable in some situations and should be discussed with a physician. Cranberry juice may be effective for preventing UTIs and is of low risk. Its effectiveness relative to the conventional approach with prescription antibiotics has not been investigated.

Conventional treatment with antibiotics should be used to treat UTIs, because the effectiveness of CAM approaches for treating UTIs, including cranberry juice, is not established. Also, people with MS and UTIs should attempt to eliminate the infection as quickly as possible, because the infection may worsen neurological symptoms.

It is important to undergo a medical evaluation for urinary incontinence. Because CAM therapies have not been extensively studied, it is important to consider conventional therapy first in this area. Multiple CAM therapies have produced promising results for urinary incontinence:

- Acupuncture
- Biofeedback
- Cooling
- Exercise (Kegel exercises)
- Hippotherapy
- Magnets and electromagnetic therapy
- Reflexology

Other CAM Therapies

Vitamin C is sometimes recommended for preventing and treating UTIs. However, studies do not indicate that vitamin C is effective, and it carries a theoretical risk in MS because of its immune-stimulating activity. Bearberry, or uva ursi, is also sometimes recommended for UTIs. The effectiveness and safety of this herb have not been established. In some studies, marijuana has produced beneficial effects on bladder function. However, marijuana may cause significant side effects and is illegal in most states.

Bowel Problems

Several MS-associated bowel problems occur, the most common of which is constipation. Rarely, diarrhea or incontinence may occur.

Conventional Therapy

The conventional therapy of bowel problems usually involves developing a *bowel program*, with changes in food and fluid intake and possibly treatment with medications.

Possibly Effective CAM Therapies

Low-risk therapies for constipation are psyllium seed and other herbs. A conventional medical evaluation is important for incontinence of stool. Simple conventional measures are often quite effective. If CAM therapy is considered, those that have produced promising results in limited studies are:

- Biofeedback
- Exercise
- Hippotherapy
- Massage

Colds and Flu—Prevention or Decreasing Duration

Colds and flu are of interest to people with MS because these viral infections may be associated with attacks. Any measure that prevents or decreases the duration of colds and flu may be helpful.

Conventional Therapy

Conventional medical approaches in this area include flu vaccination and recently developed flu medications (Relenza and Tamiflu). Also, infection with cold or flu viruses may be prevented by simple measures such as avoiding exposure to infected people, frequent hand washing, and avoiding touching the face with the hands.

CAM Therapies

Despite some claims, no magic CAM cure is available for colds and flu. No CAM therapy for the flu has been shown to be as effective as the medications currently available. As a result, people with MS who have flu symptoms should first consider these medications before CAM therapy.

Homeopathy is low risk but of unproven benefit in this area. A variety of supplements have produced positive results in some, but not all, studies. However, these therapies are theoretically risky for people with MS because they may stimulate the immune system and thus may potentially worsen MS. These therapies are echinacea, garlic, vitamin C, and zinc.

Coordination Problems

In MS, coordination may be impaired in the arms and legs. Several factors may contribute to incoordination, including tremor, weakness, muscle stiffness, and numbness.

Conventional Therapy

Mainstream approaches to incoordination usually involve occupational therapy measures, such as the use of special devices and compensatory techniques.

Possibly Effective CAM Therapies

Small studies in people with MS and in people with other conditions suggest that some CAM therapies may improve or compensate for incoordination. These include:

- Cooling
- Music therapy
- Pets

Other CAM Therapies

Feldenkrais is one low-risk CAM therapy claimed to be effective in this area but not well studied.

Depression

Many people with MS experience depression. This condition may be serious and, consequently, should be evaluated and treated by a physician.

Conventional Therapy

Conventional therapy for depression is definitely effective and includes antidepressant medication and psychotherapy.

Possibly Effective CAM Therapies

As mentioned, complaints of depression warrant evaluation by a conventional medical approach. For mild to moderate depression, some CAM therapies may be considered with the supervision of a physician. Two low-risk and low-cost therapies that are probably effective are:

- Exercise
- St. John's wort

Many other CAM therapies are possibly effective and of low risk. Further studies are needed to determine whether these therapies are truly effective. They include:

- Acupuncture
- Aromatherapy
- Ayurveda
- Hippotherapy
- Massage
- Meditation
- Music therapy
- Prayer
- SAMe
- Spirituality
- T'ai chi
- Therapeutic touch
- Yoga

Other CAM Therapies

Homeopathy is safe but of uncertain effectiveness for depression. One dietary supplement, 5-HTP, is possibly beneficial but also may be unsafe. DHEA is of unproven benefit and may be harmful.

Fatigue

MS-associated fatigue is common and may be quite disabling. Fatigue has multiple causes, including the MS disease process itself, depression, medication effects, and other medical conditions.

Conventional Therapy

Because of the multiple factors involved in fatigue, a physician or other health care provider should assess this symptom and determine the best treatment options. Mainstream therapy for fatigue, which is often quite effective, includes lifestyle modifications and medications.

Possibly Effective CAM Therapies

After a medical evaluation, CAM therapy may be considered for mild fatigue or for fatigue that does not respond to conventional treatment. Several CAM therapy options are possible, none of which have undergone rigorous evaluation in MS:

- Acetyl-L-carnitine
- Caffeine, including caffeine tablets, coffee, and other caffeine-containing herbs
- Cooling
- Exercise
- Magnets and electromagnetic therapy
- Prokarin
- T'ai chi
- Yoga

Other CAM Therapies

Homeopathy is a low-risk therapy for fatigue, but of uncertain effectiveness. Asian ginseng may be effective for fatigue but also may activate the immune system.

Several supplements are of uncertain benefit for fatigue and may be unsafe. These include androstenedione, DHEA, Siberian ginseng, and Spirulina.

Osteoporosis

As a result of inactivity, steroid use, limited sun exposure, and other factors, people with MS may be at risk for developing osteoporosis, a decrease in the density of bone tissue. A milder form of this same bone condition, osteopenia, also may occur.

Conventional Therapies

Mainstream therapy involves a variety of prescription medications along with calcium and vitamin D. In postmenopausal women, hormone replacement therapy also is considered.

Possibly Effective CAM Therapies

During conventional medical visits, osteoporosis and osteopenia are not always strongly considered in people with MS. Also, the use of vitamin D and calcium may not be seriously considered for people with osteopenia (a mild form of bone tissue loss) or for those with normal bone tissue and risk factors for osteoporosis. For these reasons, recognition and treatment or prevention of decreased bone density may conceivably be considered "alternative." Simple approaches that are effective, inexpensive, and safe are:

■ Exercise
■ Vitamin D and calcium

Pain—General

Pain is relatively common with MS. It may be caused by MS lesions in the nervous system or by weakness or stiffness that produce pain in the joints or muscles.

Conventional Therapy

The mainstream treatment of pain depends on its type and severity. Therapies include anti-inflammatory medications, specific medications that are effective for nerve-related pain, and physical therapy.

Possibly Effective CAM Therapies

CAM approaches may be worth considering if pain is mild or not completely alleviated by conventional approaches. Therapies that have produced promising results are:

■ Acupuncture
■ Ayurveda
■ Biofeedback
■ Guided imagery
■ Hypnosis
■ Magnets and electromagnetic therapy
■ Massage
■ Meditation
■ Music therapy
■ Therapeutic touch
■ Yoga

Other CAM Therapies

Feldenkrais and homeopathy are generally safe but are of uncertain effectiveness for MS-related pain. In some studies, marijuana has produced beneficial effects with pain. However, marijuana may cause significant adverse effects, and it is illegal in most states.

Sexual Problems

MS may cause sexual difficulties, including decreased libido, erection difficulties, and reduced genital sensation. Physical or psychological causes for these sexual problems also may be present.

Conventional Therapy

Because of the complexities in this area, conventional medical evaluation attempts first to identify the underlying problem and then to provide appropriate treatment. Conventional measures include medications, lubricants, sexual techniques, and counseling.

Possibly Effective CAM Therapies

Because sexual difficulties in MS are complicated, it is best to be evaluated by a physician or other health care provider. Few CAM therapies have been examined in this area. Cooling has produced possibly beneficial results, but further studies are needed to determine whether it is definitely effective.

Other CAM Therapies

Yohimbe, an herbal supplement, may be beneficial for erectile difficulties, but it also may produce significant side effects. DHEA, another supplement, is claimed to be helpful for sexual difficulties. It is of unclear benefit, however, and may lead to adverse effects.

Sleep Problems

Sleep problems are more likely to occur in people with MS than in the general population. Stiffness and spasms may contribute to sleeping difficulties, and lack of sleep may cause fatigue. Many other factors also are related to sleep difficulties in people with MS.

Conventional Therapy

A conventional medical evaluation for a sleep problem initially involves determining its underlying cause. Treatment includes medications that promote sleep and medications and other measures that improve symptoms that may interfere with sleep, such as spasms.

Possibly Effective CAM Therapies

A mainstream medical evaluation should be obtained for sleeping problems. CAM therapies may be considered for mild sleeping difficulties or those that are not fully responsive to mainstream measures. CAM treatments with possible effectiveness in this area are:

- Acupuncture
- Biofeedback
- Exercise
- Hypnosis
- Meditation
- Valerian

Other CAM Therapies

Homeopathy is a low-risk approach of uncertain effectiveness for sleep problems. Several supplements are promoted for insomnia. As discussed elsewhere in this book, melatonin may be beneficial, but in people with MS it is associated with a theoretical risk because of its immune-stimulating activity. 5-HTP, another supplement, has unclear effectiveness for insomnia and may be harmful. Marijuana has produced positive results in some studies. However, it also may cause significant side effects and is illegal in most states. Kava kava sometimes is recommended for insomnia, but most studies of this herb have actually only evaluated its effectiveness for anxiety. In any case, kava kava should be avoided because of possible liver toxicity.

Spasticity (Muscle Stiffness)

MS may cause spasticity, or muscle stiffness. This usually is due to MS-associated nervous-system injury. MS also may produce spasms, a related symptom characterized by brief, strong muscle contractions.

Conventional Therapy

The mainstream approach to spasticity frequently begins with simple exercise techniques developed by a physical therapist. Medications such as lioresal (Baclofen) and tizanidine (Zanaflex) often are used. Injections of medications or other specialized therapeutic techniques are used for severe spasticity that does not respond to treatment with medications.

Possibly Effective CAM Therapies

No CAM therapies have been studied extensively for spasticity. It is unlikely that any form of CAM will relieve moderate or severe spasticity; conventional therapy should definitely be used. CAM therapy may be worth considering for spasticity that cannot be fully managed with conventional therapy or for mild spasticity. Low-risk therapies that have produced promising results in small studies include:

- Ayurveda
- Biofeedback
- Cooling
- Exercise
- Hippotherapy
- Magnets and electromagnetic therapy
- Massage
- Reflexology
- T'ai chi
- Yoga

Other CAM Therapies

Pilates is a low-risk therapy claimed to be effective in this area, but it has not been formally studied. Marijuana has produced positive results in small studies. However, it also may produce adverse effects, and it is illegal in most states.

Thinking (Cognitive) Problems

MS may affect the brain in such a way that thinking difficulties develop. MS may impair memory and the ability to perform multiple tasks.

Conventional Therapy

A conventional approach to cognitive problems includes evaluation of cognitive function and assessment for depression or anxiety, both of which may affect thinking processes. Treatment may involve rehabilitation in identified areas of weakness and appropriate therapy for significant depression or anxiety. Prescription medications for Alzheimer's disease are sometimes used to attempt to improve MS-associated cognitive difficulties.

Possibly Effective CAM Therapies

Limited studies in people with MS have indicated beneficial effects with:

- Cooling
- *Ginkgo biloba*
- Magnets and electromagnetic therapy

Further studies are needed to evaluate whether these therapies are definitely effective.

Other CAM Therapies

Another CAM therapy, music therapy, is associated with minimal risks and has produced beneficial cognitive effects in other groups of people, especially the elderly.

Walking Problems

MS often causes walking difficulties. This may be the result of impaired leg function caused by weakness, stiffness, clumsiness, or numbness.

Conventional Therapy

The evaluation and treatment of walking difficulties generally is done by physical therapists. Treatment usually involves an individualized physical therapy program. Other measures include medications for spasticity and assistive devices, such as braces, canes, and walkers.

Possibly Effective CAM Therapies

It may be reasonable to consider CAM for walking difficulties that are mild or do not respond well to mainstream approaches. In limited studies, multiple low-risk CAM therapies have produced promising beneficial effects for people with walking difficulties:

- Cooling
- Exercise
- Hippotherapy
- Magnets and electromagnetic therapy
- Music therapy
- Pets
- T'ai chi

Other CAM Therapies

Feldenkrais is a low-risk therapy claimed to be effective for walking difficulties, but it has not been well studied.

Weakness

The nervous-system injury in MS frequently produces weakness of the arms and legs. A lack of physical activity also may produce weakness through a process of physical deconditioning.

Conventional Therapy

Conventional medicine relies on physical therapists to determine which muscles are weak and to develop an individualized exercise program to strengthen these muscles.

Possibly Effective CAM Therapies

CAM therapies should not be relied on for severe weakness. It may be reasonable to use CAM for mild weakness or for weakness that does not respond significantly to conventional therapy. Limited studies in MS and other conditions indicate that several therapies may improve or compensate for weakness:

- Acupuncture
- Cooling
- Exercise
- Hippotherapy
- Pets
- T'ai chi

Other CAM Therapies

Creatine and the Pilates method are two low-risk CAM therapies that theoretically might be effective for weakness but are relatively unstudied. One small study of creatine in MS did not demonstrate increased strength. Androstenedione, a supplement that has been claimed to increase strength, has not been shown to be effective and may actually be harmful.

Multiple (Five or More) Symptoms

People with MS may experience a variety of symptoms associated with the disease. These symptoms may be physical, such as muscle stiffness, weakness, or walking difficulties; emotional, such as depression or anxiety; or "invisible," such as fatigue.

Conventional Therapy

Conventional therapy usually is prescribed for one specific symptom. As a result, not many conventional MS therapies are effective for multiple symptoms. Physical therapy and occupational therapy may potentially improve function in a variety of areas, and some medications, such as antidepressant and anticonvulsant medications, may be effective for several different symptoms.

Possibly Effective CAM Therapies

In contrast to the symptom-specific or disease-specific approach of conventional medicine, CAM includes a number of therapies touted as being effective for many diseases or many symptoms. Although many of these multiple-symptom therapies do not live up to their claims, some CAM therapies for MS appear to be of low risk and have produced promising results for multiple symptoms:

- Acupuncture
- Biofeedback
- Cooling
- Exercise
- Hippotherapy
- Magnets and electromagnetic therapy
- Massage
- Music therapy
- T'ai chi

Other CAM Therapies

Some CAM therapies are claimed to be effective for multiple symptoms but have not been studied or are of uncertain effectiveness. Those that are of low risk include homeopathy, prayer, and spirituality.

Multiple CAM therapies are unstudied or unlikely to be beneficial; at the same time, they are possibly unsafe, expensive, or labor-intensive. Because of these concerns, these therapies should be fully investigated and well understood before use: calcium EAP, Candida (yeast) therapy, chelation therapy, dental amalgam removal, DHEA, hyperbaric oxygen, Prokarin, and toxin avoidance.

Appendix

*Summary of the Effects of Popular Dietary Supplements**

Alfalfa: Immune-stimulating

Aloe: May interact with steroids, possible toxic effects with oral use

Alpha-lipoic acid: Promising studies in animal model of MS, human studies are underway

Androstenedione: Multiple possible toxic effects

Ashwagandha: Ayurvedic herb that is sometimes recommended for MS, may be immune-stimulating

Asian ginseng: No definite therapeutic effects; possibly immune-stimulating; may interact with steroids; may inhibit blood clotting; may interact with warfarin (Coumadin)

Astragalus: Possibly immune-stimulating

Barberry: Possibly sedating

Bayberry: May interact with steroids

Bearberry: Also known as uva ursi; possible liver toxicity

Bee pollen: No definite therapeutic effects; rarely causes severe allergic reactions

Beta-carotene: *See* Vitamin A

Bissy nut: *See* Cola nut

Black currant seed oil: Contains gamma-linolenic acid; unknown safety, especially for long-term use

---

*This summary provides limited information about popular supplements. See the index for a more complete listing of popular and nonpopular supplements covered in this book. See the text itself for more detailed information on supplements.

Blue-green algae: *See* Spirulina

Borage seed oil: Possibly immune-suppressing; contains gamma-linolenic acid; possible liver toxicity; may cause seizures

Caffeine: Improves mental alertness; may irritate urinary tract

Cat's claw: Possibly immune-stimulating

Chamomile: Possibly fatigue-producing

Chaparral: Possible liver toxicity

Cod-liver oil: Possibly immune-suppressing; contains omega-three fatty acids; may inhibit blood clotting; may interact with warfarin (Coumadin)

Coenzyme Q10: Immune-stimulating; may interact with warfarin (Coumadin)

Coffee: Contains caffeine; improves mental alertness; may irritate urinary tract

Cola nut: Also known as bissy nut; contains caffeine; improves mental alertness; may irritate urinary tract

Comfrey: Possible liver toxicity

Cranberry: Possibly effective to prevent urinary tract infections; should not be used to treat urinary tract infections

DHEA: Variable immune effects; possible adverse effects

Echinacea: Not definitely effective for treating viral infections; immune-stimulating; possible liver toxicity when taken with medications that have possible liver toxicity

Ephedra: *See* Ma huang

Evening primrose oil: Possibly immune-suppressing; contains gamma-linolenic acid; may cause seizures; may inhibit blood clotting; may interact with warfarin (Coumadin)

Fish oil: Possibly immune-suppressing; contains omega-three fatty acids; less than 3 grams of EPA and DHA daily is generally safe; may inhibit blood clotting; may interact with warfarin (Coumadin)

Flaxseed oil: Possibly immune-suppressing; contains omega-three and omega-six fatty acids; greater than 45 grams daily may produce diarrhea

Garlic: Possibly immune-stimulating; may inhibit blood clotting; may interact with warfarin (Coumadin)

Germanium: Sometimes recommended for MS; no known beneficial effects for MS; may cause kidney failure and death

Ginkgo biloba: Not effective for treating MS attacks; unstudied for other uses in MS; may inhibit blood clotting; may interact with warfarin (Coumadin); may provoke seizures

Goldenseal: Possibly fatigue-producing

Guarana: Contains caffeine; improves mental alertness; may irritate urinary tract

5-HTP: Possible toxic effects

Kava kava: May cause severe liver toxicity and should be avoided; possibly effective for treating anxiety; possibly fatigue-producing

Licorice: Possibly immune-stimulating; may interact with steroids; multiple possible toxic effects

Lobelia: Multiple possible toxic effects

Ma huang: Multiple possible toxic effects, including death; may interact with steroids

Melatonin: Possibly immune-stimulating

Niacin: *See* Vitamin B$_3$

Oligomeric proanthocyanidins: Possibly immune-stimulating

Passionflower: Possibly fatigue-producing

Propolis: No definite therapeutic effects; unknown safety

Psyllium: U.S. Food and Drug Administration (FDA)-approved for constipation; should not be used by people with swallowing difficulties

Pycnogenol: Possibly immune-stimulating; safety of long-term use is unknown

Pyridoxine: *See* Vitamin B$_6$

Royal jelly: No definite therapeutic effects; may rarely provoke asthma and cause severe allergic reactions

S-adenosylmethionine: *See* SAMe

Sage: Possibly fatigue-producing

St. John's wort: Probably effective for treating depression; possibly fatigue-producing; may interact with multiple medications, including antidepressants and antiseizure medications

SAMe: Also known as S-adenosylmethionine; possibly effective for treating depression

Saw palmetto: Possibly immune-stimulating

Selenium: Possibly immune-stimulating; greater than 400 micrograms daily may produce multiple toxic effects

Siberian ginseng: No definite therapeutic effects; immune-stimulating; possibly fatigue-producing; may inhibit blood clotting; may interact with warfarin (Coumadin)

Spirulina: Also known as blue-green algae; contains variable amounts of gamma-linolenic acid; safety of long-term use is unknown

Stinging nettle: Possibly immune-stimulating; possibly fatigue-producing; may interact with warfarin (Coumadin)

Uva ursi: *See* Bearberry

Valerian: Possibly effective for treating insomnia; possibly fatigue-producing; safety of long-term use is unknown

Vitamin A: Chemically related to beta-carotene; immune-stimulating; greater than 10,000 IU daily may produce toxic effects; may increase cancer risk in smokers

Vitamin B_3: Also known as niacin; greater than 35 milligrams daily may produce toxic effects

Vitamin B_6: Also known as pyridoxine; greater than 50 milligrams daily may produce toxic effects

Vitamin B_{12}: Effective for treating documented vitamin B_{12} deficiency

Vitamin C: Not definitely effective for treating urinary tract infections or viral infections; immune-stimulating; greater than 2,500 milligrams daily may produce toxic effects; may interact with warfarin (Coumadin)

Vitamin D: Effective for preventing and treating osteoporosis; greater than 2,000 IU daily may produce toxic effects

Vitamin E: Supplements of vitamin E may be indicated with a high intake of polyunsaturated fatty acids; immune-stimulating; greater than 1,000 IU daily may produce toxic effects; may inhibit bleeding; may interact with warfarin (Coumadin)

Vitamin K: May interact with warfarin (Coumadin)

Yohimbe or yohimbine: Multiple possible toxic effects

Zinc: Possibly immune-stimulating

$\mathcal{R}eferences$

Chapter 1: Complementary and Alternative Medicine and MS

1. Eisenberg D, Davis R, Ettner S, et al. Trends in alternative medicine use in the United States, 1990–1997. *JAMA* 1998;280:1569–1575.
2. Eisenberg D, Kessler R, Foster C, et al. Unconventional medicine in the United States. *N Engl J Med* 1993;328:246–252.
3. Barnes PM, Powell-Griner E, McFann K, et al. Complementary and alternative medicine use among adults: United States, 2002. *Adv Data* 2004;343:1–20.
4. Kessler RC, Davis RB, Foster DF, et al. Long-term trends in the use of complementary and alternative medical therapies in the United States. *Ann Intern Med* 2001;135:262–268.
5. Berkman CS, Pignotti MG, Cavallo PF, et al. Use of alternative treatments by people with multiple sclerosis. *Neurorehab Neural Repair* 1999;13:243–254.
6. Marrie RA, Hadjimichael O, Vollmer T. Predictors of alternative medicine use by multiple sclerosis patients. *Mult Scler* 2003;9:461–466.
7. Stuifbergen AK, Harrison TC. Complementary and alternative therapy use in persons with multiple sclerosis. *Rehab Nursing* 2003;28:141–147.
8. Nayak S, Matheis RJ, Schoenberger NE, et al. Use of unconventional therapies by individuals with multiple sclerosis. *Clin Rehabil* 2003;17:181–191.
9. Shinto L, Yadav V, Morris C, et al. Demographic and health-related factors associated with complementary and alternative medicine (CAM) use in multiple sclerosis. *Mult Scler* 2006;12:94–100.
10. Schwartz C, Laitin E, Brotman S, et al. Utilization of unconventional treatments by persons with MS: is it alternative or complementary? *Neurology* 1999;52:626–629.
11. Hooper KD, Pender MP, Webb PM, et al. Use of traditional and complementary medical care by patients with multiple sclerosis in South-East Queensland. *Int J MS Care* 2001;3:13–28.
12. Page SA, Verhoef MJ, Stebbins RA, et al. The use of complementary and alternative therapies by people with multiple sclerosis. *Chronic Dis Canada* 2003,24:75–79.
13. Stenager E, Stenager EN, Knudsen L, et al. The use of non-medical/alternative treatment in multiple sclerosis: a 5 year follow-up study. *Acta Neurol Belg* 1995,95:18–22.
14. Sastre-Garriga J, Munteis E, Rio J, et al. Unconventional therapy in multiple sclerosis. *Mult Scler* 2003,9:320–322.

15. Thorne S, Paterson B, Russell C, et al. Complementary/alternative medicine
     in chronic illness as informed self-care decision making. *Int Nursing Studies*
     2002,9:671–683.
16. Burnfield A. *Multiple Sclerosis: A Personal Exploration*. London: Souvenir
     Press, 1985:50.
17. Forsythe E. *Multiple Sclerosis: Exploring Sickness and Health*. London: Faber
     and Faber, 1988:50.
18. Winawer SJ. *Healing Lessons*. Boston: Little, Brown, 1998:28.
19. Winawer SJ. *Healing Lessons*. Boston: Little, Brown, 1998:57.

Chapter 2: Placebos and Psychoneuroimmunology

1. Beecher HK. The powerful placebo. *JAMA* 1955;159:1602–1606.
2. Sormani MP, Molyneaux PD, Barkhof F, et al. MRI enhancing lesion fre-
    quency from patients with MS enrolled in placebo arms of clinical trials or
    in natural history studies. *MRI* 1999;17:1236–1237.
3. Hirsch RL, Johnson KP, Camenga DL. The placebo effect during a double
    blind trial of recombinant alpha2 interferon in multiple sclerosis patients:
    immunological and clinical findings. *Neurosci* 1988;39:189–196.
4. Brown RF, Tennant CC, Dunn SM, et al. A review of stress-relapse interac-
    tions in multiple sclerosis: important features and stress-mediating and -
    moderating variables. *Mult Scler* 2005;11:477–484.
5. Mohr DC, Hart SL, Julian L, et al. Association between stressful life events
    and exacerbation in multiple sclerosis: a meta-analysis. *Br Med J* 2004;
    328:731–735.
6. Katz J. *The silent world of doctor and patient*. New York: London, Collier,
    McMillan, 1984:191.

Chapter 4: Acupuncture and Traditional Chinese Medicine

1. NIH Consensus Development Panel on Acupuncture. *JAMA* 1998;
    280:1518–1524.
2. Spoerel WE, Paty DW, Kertesz A, et al. Acupuncture and multiple sclerosis.
    CMA Journal 1974;110:751.
3. Smith MO, Rabinowitz N. Acupuncture treatment of multiple sclerosis: Two
    detailed clinical presentations. *Am J Acupuncture* 1986;14:143–146.
4. Miller RE. An investigation into the management of the spasticity experi-
    enced by some patients with multiple sclerosis using acupuncture based on
    traditional Chinese medicine. *Compl Ther Med* 1996;4:58–62.
5. Steinberger A. Specific irritability of acupuncture points as an early symptom
    of multiple sclerosis. *Am J Chinese Med* 1986;14:175–178.
6. Bowling AC, Stewart TM. Efficacy, safety, and prevalence of acupuncture use
    among a group of people with MS: a web-based survey. *Int J MS Care* 2002;
    4:95.
7. Wang Y, Hashimoto S, Ramsum D, et al. A pilot study of the use of alternative
    medicine in multiple sclerosis patients with special focus on acupuncture.
    Neurology 1999;52:A550.
8. Xi L, Zhiwen L, Huayan W, et al. Preventing relapse in multiple sclerosis
    with Chinese medicine. *J Chin Med* 2001;66:39–40.

9. Yi S, Xiaoyan L. A review on traditional Chinese medicine in prevention and treatment of multiple sclerosis. *J Trad Chinese Med* 1999;19:65–73.

Chapter 6: Aromatherapy

1. Walsh E, Wilson C. Complementary therapies in long-stay neurology in-patient settings. *Nursing Standard* 1999;13:32–35.
2. Hirsh AR. Aromatherapy: art, science, or myth? In: Weintraub MI, Micozzi M, eds. *Alternative and complementary treatment in neurologic illness*. Philadelphia: Churchill Livingstone, 2001, pp. 128–150.

Chapter 9: Bee Venom Therapy and Other Forms of Apitherapy

1. Lublin FD, Oshinsky RJ, Perreault M, et al. Effect of honey bee venom on EAE. *Neurology* 1998;50:A424.
2. Wesselius T, Heersema DJ, Mostert JP, et al. A randomized crossover study of bee sting therapy for multiple sclerosis. *Neurology* 2005;65:1764–1768.

Chapter 15: Cooling Therapy

1. Capell E, Gardella M, Leandri M, et al. Lowering body temperature with a cooling suit as symptomatic treatment for thermosensitive multiple sclerosis patients. *Ital J Neurol Sci* 1995;16:533–539.
2. Flensner G, Lindencrona C. The cooling-suit: a study of ten multiple sclerosis patients' experience in daily life. *J Adv Nurs* 1999;29:1444–1453.
3. NASA/MS Cooling Study Group. A randomized controlled study of the acute and chronic effects of cooling therapy for MS. *Neurology* 2003;60:1955–1960.

Chapter 16: Craniosacral Therapy

1. Upledger JE. *CranioSacral therapy*. Berkeley, CA: North Atlantic Books, 2001:88–89.
2. Greenman PE, McPartland JM. Cranial findings and iatrogenesis from craniosacral manipulation in patients with traumatic brain syndrome. *J Am Osteopath Assoc* 1995;95:182–188,191–192.

Chapter 18: Diets and Fatty-Acid Supplements

1. Swank RL. Multiple sclerosis: twenty years on low fat diet. *Arch Neurol* 1970;23:460–474.
2. Swank RL, Dugan BB. Effect of low saturated fat diet in early and late cases of multiple sclerosis. *Lancet* 1990;336:37–39.
3. Swank RL, Goodwin J. Review of MS patient survival on a Swank low saturated fat diet. *Nutrition* 2003;16:161–162.
4. Miller JHD, Zilkha KJ, Langman MJS, et al. Double-blind trial of linoleate supplementation of the diet in multiple sclerosis. *Br Med J* 1973;1:765–768.
5. Bates D, Fawcett PRW, Shaw DA, et al. Polyunsaturated fatty acids in treatment of acute remitting multiple sclerosis. *Br Med J* 1978;2:1390–1391.
6. Paty DW, Cousin HK, Read S, et al. Linoleic acid in multiple sclerosis: failure to show any therapeutic benefit. *Acta Neurol Scand* 1978;58:53–58.

7.   Dworkin RH, Bates D, Millar JHD, et al. Linoleic acid and multiple sclerosis: a reanalysis of three double-blind trials. *Neurology* 1984;34:1441–1445.

8.   Bates D, Fawcett PRW, Shaw DA, et al. Trial of polyunsaturated fatty acids in non-relapsing multiple sclerosis. *Br Med J* 1977;10:932–933.

9.   Gibson Robert A, Lines David R, Neumann Mark A. Gamma linolenic acid (GLA) content of encapsulated evening primrose oil products. *Lipids* 1992;27:82–84.

10. Bates D, Cartlidge NEF, French JM, et al. A double-blind controlled trial of long chain n-3 polyunsaturated fatty acids in the treatment of multiple sclerosis. *J Neurol Neurosurg Psychiatry* 1989;52:18–22.

11. Goldberg P, Fleming MC, Picard EH. Multiple sclerosis: decreased relapse rate through dietary supplementation with calcium, magnesium and vitamin D. *Med Hypoth* 1986;21:193–200.

12. Nordvik I, Myhr KM, Nyland H, et al. Effects of dietary advice and n-3 supplementation in newly diagnosed MS patients. *Acta Neurol Scand* 2000;102:143–149.

13. Weinstock-Guttman B, Baier M, Park Y, et al. Low fat dietary intervention with omega-3 fatty acid supplementation in multiple sclerosis patients. *Prostaglandins Leukotrienes Essential Fatty Acids* 2005;73:392–404.

14. Rowland L, ed. *Merritt's Neurology*. Philadelphia: Lippincott, Williams & Wilkins, 2000:791.

15. Paty DW, Ebers GC, eds. *Multiple Sclerosis*. Philadelphia: FA Davis, 1998:510.

16. Kesselring J. *Multiple Sclerosis*. New York: Cambridge University Press, 1997:203.

17. Bates D. Lipids and multiple sclerosis. *Biochem Soc Trans* 1989;17:289–291.

Chapter 19: Enzyme Therapy

1.   Baumhackl U, Kappos L, Radue EW, et al. A randomized, double-blind, placebo-controlled study of oral hydrolytic enzymes in relapsing multiple sclerosis. *Mult Scler* 2005;11:166–168.

Chapter 20: Exercise

1.   Petajan JH, Gappmaier E, White AT, et al. Impact of aerobic training on fitness and quality of life in multiple sclerosis. *Ann Neurol* 1996;39:432–441.

Chapter 21: Feldenkrais

1.   Johnson SK, Frederick J, Kaufman M, et al. A controlled investigation of bodywork in multiple sclerosis. *J Altern Complement Med* 1999; 5:237–243.

Chapter 22: Guided Imagery

1.   Maguire BL. The effects of imagery on attitudes and moods in multiple sclerosis patients. *Alt Ther* 1996;2:75–79.

2.   Hall H, Minnes L, Olness K. The psychophysiology of voluntary immunomodulation. *Int J Neurosci* 1993;69:221–234.

Chapter 23: Herbs

1. Stewart TM, Bowling AC. A survey of issues related to fatigue among a large group of people with MS. *Int J MS Care* 2003;5:96.
2. Korwin-Piotrowska T, Nocon D, Stankowska-Chomicz A, et al. Experience of padma 28 in multiple sclerosis. *Phytother Res* 1992;6:133–136.
3. Blumenthal M, ed. *The Complete German Commission E Monographs: Therapeutic Guide to Herbal Medicines.* Austin: American Botanical Council, 1998:441.
4. Brinker F. *Herb Contraindications and Drug Interactions.* Oregon: Eclectic Medical Publishers, 1998:150–151.

Chapter 24: Hippotherapy and Therapeutic Horseback Riding

1. Hammer A, Nilsagard Y, Forsberg A, et al. Evaluation of therapeutic riding (Sweden)/hippotherapy (United States). A single-subject experimental design study replicated in eleven patients with multiple sclerosis. *Physiother Theory Prac* 2005;21:51–77.
2. MacKay-Lyons M, Conway C, Roberts W. Effects of therapeutic riding on patients with multiple sclerosis: a preliminary trial. *Proceedings of the 6th International Therapeutic Riding Congress* 1988;8:173–178.
3. Pfotenhauer M, Leyerer U, David E, et al. Hippotherapy, scientific program in Herdecke, an example. *Proceedings of the 7th International Therapeutic Riding Congress* 1991;August:46–57.

Chapter 25: Homeopathy

1. Swayne J. *Homeopathic Method: Implications for Clinical Practice and Medical Science.* New York: Churchill Livingstone, 1998:191.
2. Kleijnen J, Knipschild P, ter Riet G. Clinical trials of homoeopathy. *Br Med J* 1991;302:316–326.
3. Linde K, Clausius N, Ramirez G, et al. Are the clinical effects of homoeopathy placebo effects? A meta-analysis of placebo-controlled trails. *Lancet* 1997;350:834–843.
4. Linde K, Scholz M, Ramirez G, et al. Impact of study quality on outcome in placebo-controlled trials of homeopathy. *J Clin Epidemiol* 1999;52:631–636.
5. Shang A, Huwiler-Muntener K, Nartey L, et al. Are the clinical effects of homeopathy placebo effects? Comparative study of placebo-controlled trials of homeopathy and allopathy. *Lancet* 2005;366:726–732.

Chapter 26: Hyperbaric Oxygen

1. Fischer BH, Marks M, Reich T. Hyperbaric oxygen treatment of multiple sclerosis. A randomized, placebo-controlled, double-blind study. *N Engl J Med* 1983;308:181–186.
2. Kleijnen J, Knipschild P. Hyperbaric oxygen for multiple sclerosis: review of controlled trials. *Acta Neurol Scand* 1995;91:330–334.
3. Bennett M, Heard R. Hyperbaric oxygen therapy for multiple sclerosis. *Cochrane Database Syst Rev* 2004;(1):CD003057.

4. Neubauer RA, Neubauer V, Gottlieb SF. The controversy over hyperbaric oxygenation therapy for multiple sclerosis. *J Amer Phys Surgeons* 2005; 10:112–115.

Chapter 27: Hypnosis

1. Dane JR. Hypnosis for pain and neuromuscular rehabilitation with multiple sclerosis: case summary, literature review, and analysis of outcomes. *Int J Clin Exp Hypn* 1996;44:208–231.
2. Sutcher H. Hypnosis as adjunctive therapy for multiple sclerosis: a progress report. *Am J Clin Hypn* 1997;39:283–290.
3. Sutherland G, Andersen MB, Morris T. Relaxation and health-related quality of life in multiple sclerosis: the example of autogenic training. *J Behav Med* 2005;28:249–256.

Chapter 28: Low-Dose Naltrexone (LDN)

1. Agrawal YP. Low-dose naltrexone therapy in multiple sclerosis. *Med Hypotheses* 2005;64:721–724.

Chapter 29: Magnets and Electromagnetic Therapy

1. Nielsen JF, Sinkjaer T, Jakobsen J. Treatment of spasticity with repetitive magnetic stimulation: a double-blind placebo-controlled study. *Mult Scler* 1996;2:227–232.
2. Guseo A. Pulsing electromagnetic field therapy of multiple sclerosis by the Gyuling-Bordás device: double-blind, cross-over and open studies. *J Bioelec* 1987;6:23–35.
3. Richards TL, Lappin MS, Acosta-Urquidi J, et al. Double-blind study of pulsing magnetic field effects on multiple sclerosis. *J Alt Complement Med* 1997;3:21–29.
4. Lappin MS, Lawrie FW, Richards TL, et al. Effects of a pulsed electromagnetic therapy on multiple sclerosis fatigue and quality of life: a double-blind, placebo controlled trial. *Alt Ther* 2003;9:38–48.

Chapter 30: Marijuana

1. Zajicek J, Fox P, Sanders H, et al. Cannabinoids for treatment of spasticity and other symptoms related to multiple sclerosis (CAMS study): multicentre randomised placebo-controlled trial. *Lancet* 2003;362:1517–1526.
2. Zajicek J, Sanders HP, Wright DE, et al. Cannabinoids in multiple sclerosis (CAMS) study: safety and efficacy data for 12 months follow up. *J Neurol Neurosurg Psych* 2005;76:1664–1669.
3. Wade DT, Makela P, Robson P, et al. Do cannabis-based medicinal extracts have general or specific effects on symptoms in multiple sclerosis: a double-blind, randomized, placebo-controlled study on 160 patients. *Mult Scler* 2004;10:434–441.

Chapter 31: Massage

1. Hernandez-Reif M, Field T, Field T, et al. Multiple sclerosis patients benefit from massage therapy. *J Bodywork Movement Ther* 1998;2:168–174.

2. Brouwer B, de Andrade VS. The effects of slow stroking on spasticity in patients with multiple sclerosis: a pilot study. *Physiother Theory Pract* 1995;11:13–21.
3. Walsh E, Wilson C. Complementary therapies in long-stay neurology in-patient settings. *Nursing Standard* 1999;13:32–35.
4. Forsythe E. *Multiple Sclerosis: Exploring Sickness and Health.* London: Faber and Faber, 1988:129.

Chapter 32: Meditation

1. Mandel Allan R, Keller Sandra M. Stress management in rehabilitation. *Arch Phys Med Rehabil* 1986;67:375–379.
2. Smith GR, McKenzie JM, Marmer DJ, et al. Psychologic modulation of the human immune response to *Varicella zoster. Arch Intern Med* 1985;145: 2110–2112.

Chapter 33: Music Therapy

1. Schmid W, Aldridge D. Active music therapy in the treatment of multiple sclerosis patients: a matched control study. *J Music Ther* 2004;61:225–240.
2. Lengdobler H, Kiessling WR. Group music therapy in multiple sclerosis: initial report of experience. *Psychother Psychosom Med Psychol* 1989;39:369–373.
3. Wiens ME, Reimer MA, Guyn HL. Music therapy as a treatment method for improving respiratory muscle strength in patients with advanced multiple sclerosis: a pilot study. *Rehabil Nurs* 1999;24:74–80.

Chapter 34: Pets

1. Dossey L. The healing power of pets: a look at animal-assisted therapy. *Alt Ther* 1997;3:8–16.

Chapter 35: Pilates Method and the Physicalmind Method

1. Hutchinson MR, Tremain L, Christiansen J, et al. Improving leaping ability in elite rhythmic gymnasts. *Med Science Sports Ex* 1998;30:1543–1547.
2. Segal NA, Hein J, Basford JR. The effects of Pilates training on flexibility and body composition: an observational study. *Arch Phys Med Rehab* 2004;85:1977–1981.

Chapter 36: Prayer and Spirituality

1. Bryd RC. Positive therapeutic effects of intercessory prayer in a coronary care unit population. *South Med J* 1988;81:826–829.
2. Roberts L, Ahmed I, Hall S. Intercessory prayer for the alleviation of ill health. *Cochrane Collab Cochrane Library* 2002;Issue 4.
3. Astin JA, Harkness E, Ernst E. The efficacy of 'distant healing': a systematic review of randomized trials. *Ann Intern Med* 2000;132:903–910.

Chapter 37: Prokarin

1. Gillson G, Wright JV, Ballasiotes G. Transdermal histamine in multiple sclerosis. Part 1: Clinical experience. *Alt Med Rev* 1999;4:424–428.

2.   Gillson G, Richards TL, Wright JV, Smith RB, Wright, JV. A double-blind pilot study of the effect of Prokarin on fatigue in multiple sclerosis. *Mult Scler.* 2002 8:30–35.

Chapter 38: Reflexology

1.   Joyce M, Richardson R. Reflexology can help MS. *Int J Alt Compl Med* 1997;July:10–12.
2.   Siev-Ner I, Gamus D, Lerner-Geva L, et al. Reflexology treatment relieves symptoms of multiple sclerosis: a randomized controlled study. *Mult Scler* 2003;9:356–361.

Chapter 39: T'ai Chi

1.   Husted C, Pham L, Hekking A, et al. Improving quality of life for people with chronic conditions: the example of t'ai chi and multiple sclerosis. *Alt Ther* 1999;5:70–74.
2.   Mills M, Allen J. Mindfulness of movement as a coping strategy in multiple sclerosis. A pilot study. *Gen Hosp Psych* 2000;22:425–431.

Chapter 40: Therapeutic Touch

1.   Payne MB. The use of therapeutic touch with rehabilitation clients. *Rehabil Nursing* 1989;14:69–72.
2.   Rosa L, Rosa E, Sarner L, et al. A close look at therapeutic touch. *JAMA* 1998;279:1005–1010.
3.   Long R, Bernhardt P, Evans W. Perception of conventional sensory cues as an alternative to the postulated 'human energy field' of therapeutic touch. *Sci Rev Alt Med* 1999;3:53–61.

Chapter 42: Tragerwork

1.   Witt PL, MacKinnon J. Trager psychophysical integration. A method to improve chest mobility of patients with chronic lung disease. *Phys Ther* 1986;66:214–217.
2.   Foster KA, Liskin J, Cen S, et al. The Trager approach in the treatment of chronic headache : a pilot study. *Alt Ther Health Med* 2004;10:40–46.
3.   Dyson-Hudson TA. Acupuncture and Trager psychophysical integration in the treatment of wheelchair user's shoulder pain in individuals with spinal cord injury. *Arch Phys Med Rehabil* 2001;82:1038.

Chapter 43: Vitamins, Minerals, and Other Nonherbal Supplements

1.   Mai J, Sorensen PS, Hansen JC. High dose antioxidant supplementation to MS patients. *Biol Trace Elem Res* 1990;24:109–117.
2.   Goldberg P, Fleming MC, Picard EH. Multiple sclerosis: decreased relapse rate through dietary supplementation with calcium, magnesium and vitamin D. *Med Hypoth* 1986;21:193–200.

3. Fleming JO, Hummel AL, Beinlich BR, et al. Vitamin D treatment of relapsing-remitting multiple sclerosis (RRMS): a MRI-based pilot study. *Neurology* 2000;54:A338.

4. Wingerchuk DM, Lesaux J, Rice GPA, et al. A pilot study of oral calcitriol (1,25-dihydroxyvitamin D3) for relapsing-remitting multiple sclerosis. *J Neurol Neurosurg Psych* 2005;76:1294–1296.

5. Kira J, Tobimatus S, Goto I. Vitamin B_{12} metabolism and massive-dose methyl vitamin B_{12} therapy in Japanese patients with multiple sclerosis. *Int Med* 1994;33:82–86.

6. Loder C, Allawi J, Horrobin DF. Treatment of multiple sclerosis with lofepramine, L-phenylalanine, and vitamin B_{12}: mechanism of action and clinical importance: roles of the locus coeruleus and central noradrenergic systems. *Med Hyp* 2002;59:594–602.

7. Wade DT, Young CA, Chaudhuri KR, Davidson DLW. A randomized placebo controlled exploratory study of vitamin B_{12}, lofepramine, and L-phenylalanine (the "Cari Loder regime") in the treatment of multiple sclerosis. *J Neurol Neurosurg Psych* 2002;73:246–249.

8. Tomassini V, Pozzilli C, Onesti E, et al. Comparison of the effects of acetyl-L-carnitine and amantadine for the treatment of fatigue in multiple sclerosis: results of a pilot, randomised, double-blind, crossover trial. *J Neurol Sci* 2004;218:103–108.

9. Marracci GH, Jones RE, McKeon GP, et al. Alpha lipoic acid inhibits T cell migration into the spinal cord and suppresses and treats experimental autoimmune encephalomyelitis. *J Neuroimmunol* 2002;131:104–114.

10. Yadav V, Marracci G, Lovera J, et al. Lipoic acid in multiple sclerosis: a pilot study. *Mult Scler* 2005;11:159–165.

11. Lambert CP, Archer RL, Carrithers JA, et al. Influence of creatine monohydrate ingestion on muscle metabolites and intense exercise capacity in individuals with multiple sclerosis. *Arch Phys Med Rehabil* 2003;84:1206–1210.

12. Zhang GX, Yu S, Gran B, et al. Glucosamine abrogates the acute phase of experimental autoimmune encephalomyelitis by induction of Th2 response. *J Neuroimmunol* 2005;175:7202–7208.

13. Scott GS, Spitsin SV, Kean RB, et al. Therapeutic intervention in experimental allergic encephalomyelitis by administration of uric acid precursors. *Proc Natl Acad Sci* 2002;99:16303–16308.

14. Spitsin S, Hooper DC, Leist T, et al. Inactivation of peroxynitrite in multiple sclerosis patients after oral administration of inosine may suggest possible approaches to therapy of the disease. *Mult Scler* 2001;7:313–319.

15. Platten M, Ho PP, Yousseff S, et al. Treatment of autoimmune neuroinflammation with a synthetic tryptophan metabolite. *Science* 2005;310:850–855.

Chapter 44: Yoga

1. Oken BS, Kishiyama S, Zajdel D, et al. Randomized controlled trial of yoga and exercise in multiple sclerosis. *Neurology* 2004;62:2058–2064.

Index

The letter *t* following a page number refers to a table on that page.